WHAT YOU MUST KNOW ABOUT
AGE-RELATED MACULAR DEGENERATION

HOW YOU CAN PREVENT, STOP, OR REVERSE AMD

JEFFREY ANSHEL, OD
LAURA STEVENS, M.Sci

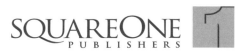
SQUAREONE
PUBLISHERS

The information and advice contained in this book are based upon the research of the authors, and are not intended as a substitute for consulting with a healthcare professional. The publisher and authors are not responsible for any adverse effects or consequences resulting from the use of any of the suggestions presented in the book. All matters pertaining to your physical health, including your diet, should be supervised by a healthcare professional who can provide medical care that is tailored to meet individual needs.

COVER DESIGNER: Jeannie Tudor
TYPESETTER: Gary A. Rosenberg
IN-HOUSE EDITOR: Joanne Abrams

Square One Publishers
115 Herricks Road
Garden City Park, NY 11040
(516) 535-2010 * (877) 900-BOOK
www.squareonepublishers.com

Library of Congress Cataloging-in-Publication Data
Names: Anshel, Jeffrey, author. | Stevens, Laura J., 1945- author.
Title: What you must know about age-related macular degeneration : how you can prevent, stop, or reverse AMD / Jeffrey Anshel, OD, Laura Stevens, M.Sci.
Description: Garden City Park, NY : Square One Publishers, [2018] | Includes bibliographical references and index.
Identifiers: LCCN 2018002000 (print) | LCCN 2018002673 (ebook) | ISBN 9780757054495 | ISBN 9780757004490 (paperback) | ISBN 9780757054495 (ebook)
Subjects: LCSH: Retinal degeneration. | Eye—Aging.
Classification: LCC RE661.D3 (ebook) | LCC RE661.D3 A57 2018 (print) | DDC 617.7/35—dc23
LC record available at https://lccn.loc.gov/2018002000

Printed in the United States of America

10   9   8   7   6   5   4   3   2   1

Contents

PART FOUR

Living Successfully with Macular Degeneration

To my beloved mother and dear friend,
Phyllis Galey.

–LS

To all patients and family members who are
dealing with a macular degeneration diagnosis.
My hope is that we will be able to not just manage
this disease but stop or prevent it from ever
challenging our vision and lifestyle.

–JA

Preface

Laura's Story

My first experience with age-related macular degeneration occurred when my mother struggled with the disorder. Although she never complained and tried to pretend that she wasn't losing her sight, it eventually became apparent that she was. Once, my family and I were visiting her and my father, and we planned to watch a televised horse race together. Before she joined us in the living room, we watched the end of a TV medical drama. When my mother walked into the room, she stared at the four doctors in white uniforms on the screen and said, "Oh, there are the horses!" It was then we realized the severity of her vision issues. When she couldn't read menus in restaurants, she just ordered whatever my father ordered. AMD was greatly affecting her life.

Years later, I began to regularly visit a lady in a nursing home as part of my church's outreach ministry. When I first met the lady, I asked her how she was, and she grimly replied, "I sit, I eat, I sleep!" My friend had advanced AMD and could see only my shoes and socks with any clarity. She was in the nursing facility because her impaired vision prevented her from caring for herself, and now, because of her disability, she could not participate in most of the facility's activities. For both my mother and my friend, AMD was a game changer.

Four years ago, I was diagnosed with AMD by an ophthalmologist in Lafayette, Indiana. He said that other than taking the AREDS2 formula—the over-the-counter vitamin supplement carried in all drugstores—I should use UV- and blue light-resistant sunglasses outdoors and follow a "nutritious diet," which he did not explain further. There was nothing else I could do.

I'm a fighter, and I couldn't sit around and wait for my vision to decline as I had watched my mother's and friend's vision worsen over time. Instead, I saw an expert, an internationally known ophthalmologist in Indianapolis. He diagnosed "familial drusen" in my left eye—the right eye was not affected—and said that the condition might not progress at all. However, a year later, I noticed that my vision was worsening and I went to see him again. This time, he diagnosed AMD in both eyes. Although he worked part-time for a pharmaceutical company, where he hoped to develop treatments for AMD, he was very discouraging about the available options. All I could do was take AREDS, eat a nutritious diet, and wear sunglasses—which I was already doing. I asked about other nutrients and any future drugs in the pipeline. He said, "No other nutrients have been found to be helpful. There are no promising drugs on the immediate horizon. I'm sorry!"

Needless to say, I was scared. I was not, however, ready to accept an inevitable decline in function. In the middle 1990s, I had received my master's degree in Nutrition Science from Purdue University, and since that time, I had worked as a research associate there. I knew how to search medical literature, and because of my education in biochemistry and nutrition, I could read and understand the articles I found. So I turned my attention to learning if any nutrients other than those used in the AREDS study showed promise. Surprisingly, I found quite a few studies in which additional nutrients had not only slowed the development of AMD, but actually improved vision. I was excited!

At about the same time, my doctor in New York City, whom I had seen since 1986 for chronic fatigue syndrome, urged me to consult an herbalist. Soon, I began to learn more about herbal supplements for both my fatigue and my vision. We started to try various preparations, and I was thrilled when the vision in my left eye began to function better. I bought an eye chart so that I could track my vision and note improvements or setbacks. Every day, I also checked my Amsler Grid (see page 23) as instructed by my doctor. Maybe the scientist in me led me to document my progress.

I was hoping that my regimen of supplements would at least allow me to maintain my vision, but it did even more. When I started, I could read the top two lines of the eye chart with my left eye wearing my glasses. Over a period of several months, I began to read more and more letters. I was so excited by the articles I had read and my own personal experience that I decided to write this book. I wanted others to know that there are many things they can do to save their vision. I hope that the lifestyle changes I share in these pages—including my supplement regimen and the Anti-AMD Diet—will help my readers just as they have helped me.

Jeff's Story

As a third-year optometry school student in the 1970s, I recall sitting in a class on eye disease. This particular class dealt with the retina and its problems, and the current topic was "drusen," which we see as yellowish-white spots scattered around the retina. The professor's comment was that these were "thickening of the membrane behind the retina." He also concluded that they were common in older patients and that there was no harm in seeing them occasionally.

Fast-forward a few years to my time in the Navy. When examining retired military personnel, I saw patients lose vision associated with the development of drusen in the center of the retina. While we knew about "age-related macular degeneration," we had no idea about the development or course of the disease. All we knew is that it was more common as people aged and it resulted in functional blindness.

Following my Navy service, I started a practice in a holistic healing center near San Diego. It was there that I was exposed to the fields of chiropractic, acupuncture, colonic hydrotherapy, meditation, massage, and a number of other alternative medical therapies. The one thing that all of these practitioners had in common was their inclusion of nutrition as part of treatment. They all valued nutrition—everyone except me, that is.

I felt that I had received a well-rounded education in optometry school—mine was considered one of the oldest and best schools in the country—but there had been no mention of nutrition at any level. Thus, influenced by other practitioners, I began an independent study of nutrition and eye health. In the beginning, I would tell people that I emphasized nutrition for vision, and their response was, "What, just eat carrots, right?" Apparently, I had a lot of work to do to educate the public about the importance of a good diet.

Unfortunately, at that time, there had not been much research into eye nutrition. People did not realize that the eyes are an integral part of the body—especially, the brain. My work centered on the connection of nutrition to basic human physiology. In other words, if something was good for a particular body function, it was likely good for the eyes, as well. While I tried to convey these concepts to local practitioners and my patients, there was still no national exposure to these concepts.

That changed in 2001, when a study from the National Eye Institute showed that a few nutrients (specifically, antioxidants and zinc) slowed the progression of macular degeneration. This began the public's acceptance of nutrition as a potential treatment for eye disorders. At the time, I became acquainted with the CEO of an eye supplement company, who dedicated her life to teaching eye-care professionals about various eye conditions and how they could be resolved through nutritional means. I soon realized that although the treatment of eye disorders through supplements was important, eye-care professionals were now receiving information that was filtered through supplement manufacturers and was typically skewed to support their particular products. I discussed this concern with a few colleagues, and we decided to form the Ocular Nutrition Society (ONS). The mission of the ONS was to provide leadership, education, advice, and guidance to eye-care and other health care professionals and consumers regarding the role of nutritional support in vision and eye health. The ONS supported evidence-based analysis concerning nutritional influences on eyes and systemic disease.

For six years, I devoted my time to the ONS and saw the eye-care field—including both ophthalmology and, to a larger degree, optometry—begin to learn about the use of nutrition and nutritional supplements to support both eye health and general well-being. I then decided to get back to my roots as a practitioner. Relocating my practice to my home town, I directed my energy toward treating patients on a personal level. My focus remains on nutrition, and I have been rewarded by seeing the difference I can make in the lives (and eyesight) of my patients. It is my hope that my coauthor, Laura Stevens, and I can offer our readers insight, guidance, and encouragement as they work to maintain their eyesight through proven dietary and lifestyle modifications.

$\mathcal{I}$ntroduction

As far back as Hippocrates, who advised "Let food be thy medicine," health experts have known that diet can have a great influence on physical well-being. But for a long time, most people—doctors included—did not view nutrition as being a critical element in the maintenance of good vision. That changed in 2001, when results of the Age-Related Eye Disease Study (AREDS) were published, clearly demonstrating that selected nutrients can slow the progression of age-related macular degeneration (AMD), the leading cause of vision loss in people age fifty and over. This research and the follow-up study, known as AREDS2, convinced a great many eye-care providers and their patients that supplements can improve eye health.

Although the AREDS2 formula was found to slow the progression of age-related macular degeneration, it was not found to prevent, stop, or reverse AMD, nor did it help people in the earliest stages of the disease. So when author Laura Stevens was diagnosed with this disorder, she was told by her doctor that other than taking the AREDS formula and wearing eye-protective sunglasses, there was nothing she could do to change AMD's course. Fortunately, Laura, a medical researcher at Purdue University, refused to stand by helplessly as her vision declined. Instead, she searched medical literature for studies that explored the relationship between nutrition and

1

macular degeneration. She soon found that additional nutrients could not only slow the development of this disorder but actually improve vision. The idea for this book was born when Laura's nutritional supplement regimen, enhanced diet, and other lifestyle changes began to bear fruit, and Laura realized that she was experiencing better vision and greater eye health.

Written by Laura Stevens and Jeffrey Anshel, a doctor of optometry, *What You Must Know About Age-Related Macular Degeneration* guides you in using nutritional supplements, diet, and lifestyle modifications such as exercise to help prevent, halt, or even reverse the progression of AMD. The book is based on the most recent scientific research and is supported by Laura's real-life endeavor to treat her own AMD and Jeffrey's years of experience helping patients manage eye disorders through both conventional and alternative means.

Part One of this book focuses on understanding the basics of vision and macular degeneration. Chapter 1 begins by explaining the anatomy of the eye and how the different structures work together to allow you to see an image. Included is a look at the eye structures that are specifically affected by macular degeneration.

Chapter 2 takes a close look at AMD—what it is, how it can start, and how it can progress. The chapter also discusses how AMD is diagnosed, monitored, and treated by both conventional and alternative medicine, providing the knowledge you need to better communicate with your doctor and make informed decisions about treatment.

Extensive studies have revealed the risk factors—including environmental, genetic, and lifestyle-related elements—that play a role in the development of AMD. Although some of these variables, such as age and gender, cannot be changed, you'll find that a number can (and should) be modified, enabling you to take steps to safeguard and even improve your vision. Chapter 3 explores these risk factors, while Chapter 4 focuses on one of the most common of these factors, metabolic syndrome.

As you know, the AREDS study proved that nutritional supplements are effective in the treatment of AMD. Just as important, research has shown that additional supplements can have an impact on eye health. Part Two focuses on the important topic of AMD and supplementation.

Chapter 5 looks at the AREDS trials, which provided the clinical evidence that specific supplements help protect the eyes from AMD. The nutritional approach based on the AREDS formula is now the most widely accepted means of combating this disorder.

Chapter 6 focuses on supplements that are derived from plants. Included are botanical preparations that have been specifically shown to prevent, slow, or reverse AMD, as well as plant-based supplements that have properties which can improve eye health. In addition to the discussions of specific supplements, this chapter provides basic information about the different forms in which herbal preparations can be found and guides you in using them wisely and effectively.

Chapter 7, which concludes Part Two, provides a comprehensive examination of the many vitamins, minerals, essential fatty acids, and other nutrients that you need to protect your eyes, and especially your retina. A handy table details recommended dosage as well as important considerations for usage.

Research conducted all over the world has indicated that, in addition to key nutritional supplements, a good diet is essential to eye health, just as it is essential to good health in general. The important topic of macular degeneration and your diet is explored in Part Three.

The standard Western diet is packed with foods that promote hardening of the arteries, heart disease, diabetes, and other conditions that contribute to age-related macular degeneration. Clearly, it is important to avoid the foods that are known to damage the human body. With a focus on macular degeneration and the conditions associated with it, Chapter 8 begins the discussion of diet by clearly explaining what you should *not* put on your plate. Here, you'll learn about the foods that can compromise your health so that you can either avoid them or greatly limit their use as a means of protecting your vision.

What makes a food healthy? That is the subject of Chapter 9, which begins our exploration of healthier foods by looking at the dietary components—fiber, protein, and more—that play a crucial role in maintaining vision.

Once you have learned about the nutritional components that are important for eye health, you're ready to learn about the delicious foods that contain these nutrients. Chapter 10 provides informative discussions about the many foods that should have an important place in your Anti-AMD Diet.

By the end of Chapter 10, you will know all the basics of an eye-healthy diet, but you still may wonder how you can put these dietary principles into practice. Chapter 11 shows the way by first reviewing the fundamentals of an eye-healthy diet, and then offering a number of sample menus that take the guesswork out of creating wholesome meals and snacks. Included are invaluable tips for dining out so that you can enjoy nourishing, health-promoting meals even when you're away from home.

Although diet and nutritional supplements are essential to fighting macular degeneration, there are other steps you can take to lower your risk of AMD. That's why Part Four begins with a chapter that explores the simple lifestyle modifications—such as quitting smoking, getting regular exercise, and protecting your eyes from damaging blue light—that can help you avoid or slow AMD. Finally, for those readers who are already affected by macular degeneration, the last chapter of the book is a guide to the many tools that can help you make the most of the vision that remains. Armed with the right devices and techniques, even people with advanced AMD can often participate in those activities that they need to perform as well as those that provide enjoyment.

Everyone has the ability to lead a healthier life, and this book looks at the simple steps you can take to safeguard your eye health, halt or reverse the progression of age-related macular degeneration, and maybe even improve your overall well-being. Just remember that Rome wasn't built in a day, and neither is an eye-protective lifestyle. Over time, the small changes that you begin to implement today will pay off. There is no more important investment than the investment you make in your health.

Part One

The Basics of Macular Degeneration

1

How Your Eyes Work

If you're like most people, you take your eyes and your sense of sight for granted—that is, until you begin to have vision problems. Then you go to an eye doctor to learn what is happening. Unfortunately, the language the doctor uses to explain the problem can be a little confusing and can slow your understanding of your condition. That's why this chapter was designed to first acquaint you with the anatomy of the eye—what the different parts of the eye are, and what function each of them performs—and then provide basic information on how your eye works to produce an image. Finally, you will learn how visual acuity is measured by your eye-care provider. By the end of the chapter, you will have a clear understanding of how the components of your eye interact with one another and with your brain so that you can see.

THE ANATOMY OF YOUR EYE

The eye is a slightly asymmetrical globe that is about an inch in diameter and three inches in circumference. But don't let its seemingly simple shape and small size fool you. Sometimes described as the most complex organ in the human body, the eye has many parts that work together to complete the difficult task of providing vision.

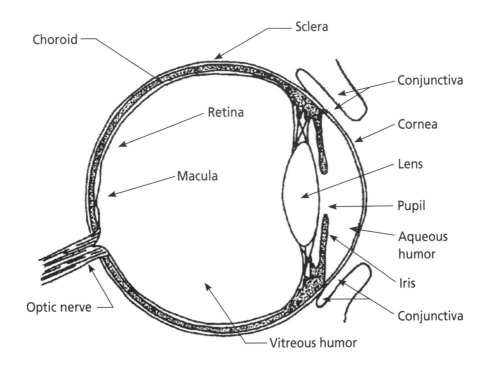

Figure 1.1. The Anatomy of the Eye.

■ THE SCLERA

The *sclera* is the dense white outer covering of the eye that is some-times known as the white of the eye. Its main purpose is to provide support and protection for the inner eye structures and to attach the eye to the six muscles that control its movement up and down and from side to side.

The cells that make up the sclera are white in color, but some blood vessels do pass through the sclera to other tissues. When these vessels become swollen or dilated, the eyes may appear bloodshot. More often, though, a reddish looking eye is the result of irritation to the *conjunctiva*, which is the thin, normally transparent membrane that covers the sclera and lines the eyelids.

■ THE CHOROID

Just inside the sclera, covering the same area as the sclera, is the *choroid*. The middle layer of the eye wall, the choroid is sandwiched between the sclera and the thin light-sensitive inner layer known as the retina. The choroid is filled with blood vessels that deliver oxygen and nutrients to the retina and to other structures found inside the eye.

■ THE CORNEA

The *cornea* is the transparent dome-shaped structure that covers the front of the eye. Together with the sclera, it makes up the outer surface of the eyeball and supports the eye's internal structures. The cornea also acts as the eye's outermost lens, functioning as a window that helps control the focusing of light into the eye. When light hits the cornea, the cornea refracts (bends) the light onto the lens. In fact, the cornea provides up to 75 percent of the eye's focusing power.

Unlike most of the structures of the body, the cornea does not contain any blood vessels. Instead, it receives nourishment from the tears that cover it and from the aqueous humor, which is directly behind it.

■ THE AQUEOUS HUMOR

The *aqueous humor* is a clear fluid that fills the small chamber between the cornea, which is in front of it, and the iris, which is behind it. This fluid holds much of the nutrition that supports the tissues in this area, including the lens. The aqueous humor flows into and out of the eye on a regular basis. When this flow is not properly controlled, potentially damaging eye pressure issues such as *glaucoma*—which is abnormally high eye pressure—can result.

■ THE IRIS AND PUPIL

The *iris* is the colored portion of the eye found in front of the lens. (See the discussion of the lens below.) This ring-shaped structure regulates the amount of light that enters the eye through the pupil, the round opening in the center of the iris. When you look directly at someone's eye, the *pupil* looks like a black spot in the middle of the colored iris.

The iris contains muscles that allow the pupil to get bigger (to open up or dilate) when there is relatively little light and get smaller (close up or constrict) when the light is bright.

■ THE LENS

Situated behind the iris, the *lens*—sometimes called the *crystalline lens*—is a transparent structure made of flexible tissue. It is biconvex in shape, meaning that both sides are thicker in the middle and thinner on the edges. The lens' elasticity allows it to change shape and focus on objects that are different distances from the eye. When the lens is stretched and thin, it can focus on distant objects. When it is thicker and more rounded, it can focus on objects that are closer. The ciliary muscles attached to the lens facilitate these shape changes. The lens is the second part of the eye that works to focus images on the retina, the first being the cornea.

A healthy lens is clear. When a lens becomes cloudy by developing a *cataract*, vision is affected.

■ THE VITREOUS HUMOR

A clear gel-like substance, the *vitreous humor* fills the large central chamber of the eye between the lens and the retina. Because the gel is firm, it helps maintain the spherical shape of the eye and supports the retina. Because it is clear, light can easily pass through it.

Unlike the aqueous humor, which flows into and out of the eye, the vitreous humor is a stagnant (unmoving) fluid. If a substance enters the gel, it remains suspended there. These suspended substances are collectively referred to as *floaters*. During the prenatal stage of development, blood vessels grow through the vitreous to feed the developing front of the eye. Just prior to birth, these blood vessels dissolve—mostly. Those cells that do not dissolve remain suspended in the middle of the vitreous. Throughout most of your life, you don't notice these small cells, but as you age, the vitreous humor softens into a fluid gel, and these cells begin to "float" around. When they move near the retina and/or macula and you look at a bright light, the floaters can cast shadows on the retina, appearing as black spots or threadlike fibers. New floaters can also form when protein fibers from the vitreous gel clump together. It is normal to see some floaters as you age, but if you suddenly begin seeing large numbers of them, it's important to contact your doctor, as this can be a sign of a detached retina or another retinal disease.

■ THE RETINA AND MACULA

The *retina* is a thin layer of tissue that lines the back of the eye. The purpose of this structure is to receive the light that is focused by the lens, convert it into neural signals, and send the signal to the brain. Human beings have what is sometimes called a "camera-type eye." The cornea and lens focus light onto the light-sensitive retina just as a camera lens focuses light onto film.

The central part of the retina, called the *macula*, offers sharp, detailed vision—the type of vision needed to thread a needle or read a book. Visual acuity is highest in the *fovea*, a small dimple found in the middle of the macula. We refer to the fovea and the macula as the *macular region*. When we discuss macular degeneration, this is the region to which we refer.

The retina is composed of several layers of cells, and one layer is embedded with specialized cells known as rods and cones. Called *photoreceptors* because they respond to light, each of these cell types has a particular function. The long, slender cells known as *rods* are responsible for vision in low levels of light, and therefore are essential to night vision. *Cones*, on the other hand, are active in higher levels of light and respond to colors, and therefore are essential to daytime vision. Our sharpest vision comes from the cones, which work under most light conditions and provide detail.

Rods and cones are not evenly distributed throughout the retina. Cones are found in greatest concentration in the area of the macula, and rods are found in the outer edges of the retina. This is why the most important detailed images are formed at the macula, while the rest of the retina provides peripheral vision—the vision at the edge of the visual field. When cones and rods receive information provided by light, they convert it into electrical signals, which are transmitted to the brain via the optic nerve.

■ THE OPTIC NERVE

Located in the back of the eye in the center of the retina, the optic nerve uses electrical impulses to transfer the visual information received by the retina to the vision centers of the brain. The retina, discussed above, contains *ganglion cells,* which are specialized nerve cells that receive signals from the rod and cone photoreceptors. The optic nerve is composed of the threadlike axons of the ganglion cells, with each optic nerve—one from each eye—containing about one million nerve fibers. The two optic nerves meet in the brain, where the electrical impulses are converted into images.

HOW THE EYE SEES

Now that you know the different parts of the eye, it's easier to understand how this organ works to transmit an image to your brain so that you can see what is around you.

Vision begins when light passes through the cornea, which starts the focusing process by bending the light so that it can enter the eye. The light then moves through the aqueous humor; through the pupil; through the lens, where the image is further focused; and then through the vitreous humor. Finally, the image is focused onto the retina, where the light stimulates the rod and cone cells. The rods and cones convert the light into electrical signals, which are sent to the visual cortex of the brain via the optic nerve. The brain then reconciles the two slightly different images it receives—one from each eye—and creates a single image. Thus, your vision is really the result of two processes: (1) the eye receiving light, and (2) the brain interpreting the signals from the eye.

MEASURING VISUAL ACUITY

Before we leave the subject of basic eye structure and function, it makes sense to take a look at *visual acuity*—the eye's ability to distinguish details and shapes of objects. If you have ever had an eye exam, your visual acuity has been tested by means of an eye chart. This test is important because it gives the doctor a starting point at which to determine the eye's function.

The visual acuity test is performed by placing an eye chart 20 feet away from the patient and asking the patient to read the chart until he reads the smallest letter which can be distinguished from that distance. The test is performed one eye at a time because vision is usually different in each eye. What most people think of as "perfect" vision is 20/20 vision, which means that you can see at 20 feet what the "optically normal" eye can see at 20 feet. If your vision is 20/40, it means that you can see at 20 feet what the normal eye can see at 40 feet. In order to see what the normal eye sees at 20 feet, you would have to move closer to the object. In short, the larger the bottom number, the poorer the sharpness of vision.

It's important to understand that having a 20/20 score on a visual acuity test does not necessarily mean that your vision is perfect. This measure indicates only the clarity of vision at a distance. Other important vision skills that contribute to visual ability include depth perception, eye coordination, peripheral vision, and color vision. Also, some people can see well at a distance but are unable to bring objects into focus when they are near to them. This can be caused by farsightedness (*hyperopia*) or loss of focusing ability (*presbyopia*).

The sharpest resolution—the clearest image—occurs at the macular region of the retina, so you can understand that the degeneration of the macula associated with AMD can have a profound effect on visual acuity. That's why a visual acuity test is just part of a thorough eye exam, which should determine not only how clearly you're seeing—whether you're near or far from the object being viewed—but also what may be affecting your ability to see well.

CONCLUSION

We have now reviewed some basic information about the anatomy of the eye and the function of the visual system. We hope that this will give you the background you need to discuss your eye condition with your doctor and understand how age-related macular degeneration (AMD) develops, progresses, and affects your vision. The next chapter specifically examines AMD—what it is, how it develops, and how it is generally treated.

2

$\mathcal{W}$hat Is Age-Related Macular Degeneration?

If you or a loved one has been diagnosed with age-related macular degeneration, or AMD, you are not alone. In 2015, it was estimated that over 1.6 million people in the United States have age-related macular degeneration, and this number is likely to double in twenty years. The macula begins to degenerate in one out of every four people over the age of sixty-five and in one out of every three people over the age of eighty. AMD is the leading cause of vision impairment in older adults in the United States.

This chapter was designed to take a close look at AMD—what it is, how it can start, and how it can progress. The chapter also discusses how AMD is diagnosed and monitored, and how it may be treated using both conventional and alternative techniques. With this knowledge, you will be able to better communicate with your eye doctor and make informed decisions regarding the management of your condition.

WHAT IS AGE-RELATED MACULAR DEGENERATION?

In Chapter 1, you learned that the macula is the area of retina that is used for detailed central vision. It is the most active area of the retina, where an abundance of cones—light- and color-sensitive cells—are located. *Age-related macular degeneration* is a progressive deterioration of the macula that has its onset after age fifty.

How does macular degeneration occur? Because there is so much activity in the retina, the cells that make up this structure must "regenerate" themselves on a regular basis. This means that the ends of the older cones (and some rods too) break off and are transported away from the retina by a waste disposal system behind the retina. With age, there can be a breakdown in this system, and deposits of yellow debris called *drusen* can accumulate in the retina.

The breakdown of this disposal system most often starts with a malfunction of the pigmented membrane behind the retina known as the *retinal pigment epithelium,* or *RPE.* This membrane is responsible for getting rid of dead cells, as well as for nourishing the fragile nerve tissue of the retina and macula and performing other functions vital to the health of the retina. When the RPE fails to dispose of the dead cells, drusen builds up along the RPE layer, which begins to block off the nutritional support of the retina. This is often accompanied by inflammation of the RPE, possibly as a reaction to the "starvation" of the rods and cones. The inflammation further prevents clearing away of cell debris, which leads to more inflammation. While it is still unknown how or why this process begins, research shows that this "inflammatory cascade" opens the doorway to AMD.

COMMON TYPES AND STAGES OF AMD

There are two general forms of AMD—dry AMD and wet AMD. The dry form includes 90 percent of cases and occurs when drusen start to accumulate beneath the macula. Vision loss from the dry form of AMD is moderate but can progress to a stage called *geographic atrophy,* in which a large portion of the retina at the back of the eyeball is dysfunctional.

The wet form of AMD accounts for the other 10 percent of cases. It occurs after the dry form, when tiny abnormal blood vessels begin to grow behind the retina in an effort to feed the oxygen-deprived retinal cells. These new abnormal blood vessels often leak blood and fluid, which damage the macula, causing rapid and severe vision loss. Everyone who has wet AMD started out with the dry form of the disorder, even if they didn't notice it. The progression of the disease has three stages.

Early AMD

At this stage, the doctor may be able to see small or medium-sized drusen scattered throughout the retina, indicating a change in the physiology of the retina. Most people do not experience vision loss in the early stage of AMD, which is why regular eye exams are important, particularly if you have more than one risk factor. (See Chapter 3 to learn about the risk factors for macular degeneration.)

Intermediate AMD

In the intermediate stage of AMD, the drusen are typically located in the macular area, and a comprehensive eye exam may detect larger drusen and/or pigment changes in the retina. There may be some vision loss at this stage, but there still may not be noticeable symptoms, especially if the loss is in only one eye.

Late AMD

This stage of AMD is characterized by multiple drusen and vision loss from macular damage. There are two forms of late AMD. The first is dry; the second is wet.

Geographic Atrophy. When the form of AMD remains dry but progresses to this stage, there is a gradual breakdown of the cells in the macula that transmit visual information to the brain, and of the tissue that supports the macula from below. These changes cause the loss of vision.

Neovascular AMD. In this form, weak blood vessels grow below the macula, where they can leak fluid and blood, causing wet AMD. This condition, in turn, results in swelling, damage, and loss or distortion of vision. The vision loss caused by neovascular AMD may be severe and occur rapidly, in contrast to the more gradual deterioration that is associated with dry AMD. It is possible to have both dry and wet AMD in the same eye.

Not every case of early AMD progresses to late AMD. When people have early AMD in one eye but no signs of the disease in the other eye, only about 5 percent develop late AMD after ten years. When they are diagnosed with early AMD in both sides, about 14 percent develop late AMD after ten years.

HOW LONG DOES AMD TAKE TO PROGRESS?

Although the early stage of AMD can be detected during a standard eye exam, many people have AMD for years before it is diagnosed and before they experience any vision problems. This makes it more

Are There Other Types of Macular Degeneration?

The early part of this chapter discusses the retinal changes that are caused by age-related macular degeneration. But deterioration of the macula can also be caused by other diseases. Below, you'll learn about three of these disorders.

Best Disease

Also called *juvenile Best disease* and *vitelliform macular dystrophy*, Best disease—like AMD—attacks the macula and is associated with the buildup of drusen. In Best disease, however, changes in the eye can begin between the ages of three and fifteen, although vision is not usually affected until later on in life. Some people with this disorder can continue to read into their forties, their fifties, or beyond. As the disease progresses, though, there is a gradual loss of central vision.

Caused by mutations in the BEST1 gene, this is an inherited eye disease that can occur in both men and women and usually affects both eyes. Currently, there is no treatment for this macular disorder, but ongoing research in gene therapy may lead to a treatment in the future.

Sorsby's Fundus Dystrophy

Like Best disease, *Sorsby's fundus dystrophy* is an inherited eye disease. Caused by a mutation in the TIMP3 gene, it is characterized by progres-

difficult to say how long it normally takes for an eye to progress from early stage to late stage AMD. In addition, when AMD occurs in only one eye, the good eye may dominate the individual's vision, masking the condition's effects on the other eye and delaying diagnosis.

We do know that in some people, AMD advances so slowly that vision loss does not occur for a long time, while in others, the disease progresses quickly and may lead to a loss of vision in both eyes or in only one eye. Generally speaking, it can take from one to ten years to progress from early-stage AMD to late-stage AMD.

Genetic testing, which requires a cheek-swab cell sample, can help predict an individual's risk for developing advanced AMD by

---

sive degeneration of the macula, with swelling, bleeding, and pigment changes. The onset typically occurs between the twenties and forties, when white and yellow spots appear (not drusen) along with the death of retinal cells. In most patients, this is followed by the growth of new blood vessels along with more bleeding. Further degeneration of the macula occurs over the years, and damage can spread from the center to the periphery of the retina. The patient often notices night blindness or difficulties in adapting to changes in light intensity before visual distortions are noticed.

At this time, there is no treatment for Sorsby's fundus dystrophy. It is likely that researchers will look into the development of therapies that can minimize the impact of the faulty gene on vision.

Stargardt Disease

Stargardt disease—also called *juvenile macular degeneration,* or STGD— is the most common form of inherited juvenile macular degeneration. It usually develops during childhood and adolescence, and like AMD, it causes the death of cells in the macula. Symptoms can include the loss of central vision, distorted vision, blind spots, blurriness, poor color vision, glare sensitivity, and difficulty in adapting to dim lighting. Side vision is usually preserved.

Currently, there is no treatment for Stargardt disease, but researchers are exploring gene, stem cell, and drug therapies.

revealing if the genes associated with this eye disorder are present. When genetic test results are evaluated along with other important risk factors—such as body mass index, smoking, and exercise—it is possible to determine the likelihood that the disease will progress over the next five years. (See Chapter 3 to learn more about AMD risk factors.)

Since the macular area is responsible for central vision only, AMD does not result in total clinical blindness, especially if only one eye is affected. However, over time, this condition can result in profound vision loss, making it difficult or impossible to read, watch television, drive, or participate in other daily activities and tasks. Therefore, it is important to do what you can to slow the progression of the disease.

HOW DO YOU KNOW IF YOU HAVE AMD?

For some people, changes in vision may be the first clue that they have macular degeneration. For many others, though, before any symptoms appear, their eye doctor detects problems with the macula during testing, and then uses follow-up tests to determine the extent to which the eye might be affected. Below, we will first look at common signs and symptoms of AMD and then briefly review the tests that are used to diagnose and monitor this disorder.

Signs and Symptoms of AMD

During the early stages of age-related macular degeneration, there may be no changes in vision. As the disorder progresses, however, symptoms of AMD may include the following.

- *Loss of contrast sensitivity.* Contrast sensitivity is the ability to distinguish a form from the background or to see subtle changes in your environment. Think of how easy it is to make out a view of a mountain during a clear day, as opposed to the same view on a foggy day. The "haze" reduces your ability to see the outline of the mountain clearly. This problem can also make it difficult to see the slight contrasts and textures in stairs or pavement.

- *Distorted vision.* The distortion of images most often occurs in the central part of the field of vision, where a grid of straight lines appears wavy, or parts of the grid may appear blank. (See the Amsler Grid on page 23.) There may also be central blind spots, shadows, or missing areas of vision.

- *Poor ability to adjust to changing levels of light.* You might notice this effect when you drive at night and have an inability to re-focus on the road after a bright headlight passes. This problem may also be apparent when you walk from a well-lighted room to a darker one, or at sunset when the light level changes quickly.

- *A decrease in visual acuity.* As AMD progresses, you may experience a drop in visual acuity of two or more levels. For instance, 20/20 vision may become 20/80 vision. (See page 12 for information on the visual acuity test.) If you have dry macular degeneration, the loss of central vision will probably be gradual. With wet macular degeneration, however, there may be a rapid onset of vision loss, likely caused by the leaking of fragile blood vessels in the macular area.

- *Impaired color perception.* You may have trouble discerning colors, especially in dim lighting conditions.

- *Impaired depth perception.* Because AMD typically occurs in one eye before the other, there is sometimes a loss of some *stereopsis*—the depth perception that results from seeing with two eyes. You may become increasingly unable to judge distances, which can make driving more hazardous and even make walking difficult.

Tests Used to Diagnose AMD

Routine eye exams sometimes reveal signs of age-related macular degeneration. The results of the visual acuity test, discussed on page 12, can show a loss of visual sharpness, but other diagnostic tools are needed to home in on the cause of the problem. Once AMD has been detected, the doctor may perform further tests to monitor its progress.

The Eye Exam

A thorough eye examination enables your eye care professional to check the inside of the eye for signs of common vision problems, including AMD. In fact, the first signs of age-related macular degeneration are usually discovered by an eye doctor during a routine eye exam.

In most cases, drops are placed in the eyes to dilate (open up) the pupils and allow more light to enter the eye. Then each eye is examined using a special magnifying lens that enables the doctor to see the tissues at the back of the eye, including the retina and macula. The exam can show the presence of AMD-related signs such as drusen deposits on the retina, pigment changes in the macula, and abnormal blood vessel development. Because AMD is a *central* retina disease, doctors often can see the problem without dilation. But dilating the pupils does allow a wider view of the retina.

Whether or not the pupils have been dilated, the doctor can use a special camera to photograph the back of the eye. This can provide more information about the health of the retina, macula, and optic nerve.

The Amsler Grid

A standard screening test for age-related macular degeneration, the Amsler Grid is used to determine whether images are distorted and/ or areas of the visual field are missing. The patient is asked to look at the grid (see Figure 2.1) and note whether the lines look wavy or otherwise indistinct and whether any parts of the grid are absent. When AMD is detected, doctors sometimes give patients copies of the grid for home testing so that they can monitor the progression of AMD by noting new or worsening distortions.

Optical Coherence Tomography (OCT)

When a doctor suspects advanced dry AMD, this noninvasive technique can be used to produce images of the retina. Optical coherence tomography (OCT) produces cross-sectional images of the retina so that the doctor can measure the different layers and their thicknesses. This can pinpoint areas of the retina that are thinning, revealing the presence of geographic atrophy. This test may also be used to assess the retina's response to AMD treatments.

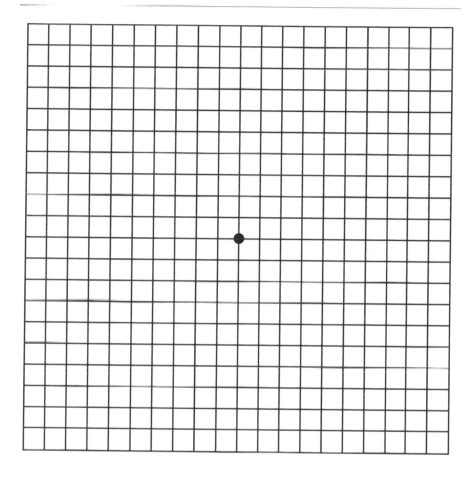

Figure 2.1. The Amsler Grid.

1. Tape this page at eye level where light is consistent and without glare.
2. Put on your reading glasses and cover one eye.
3. Fix your gaze on the center black dot.
4. Keeping your gaze fixed, try to see if any lines are distorted or missing.
5. Mark the defect on the chart.
6. TEST EACH EYE SEPARATELY.
7. If the distortion is new or has worsened, arrange to see your eye doctor at once.
8. Always keep the Amsler's Chart the same distance from your eyes each time you test.

Source: The American Macular Degeneration Foundation.

Optical Coherence Tomography Angiography (OCTA)

A newer version of OCT, discussed on page 22, called optical coherence tomography angiography, or OCTA, is also a noninvasive technique. It uses motion-contrast imaging to generate an image of blood flow down to the capillary level in a matter of seconds. Still expensive and not yet employed by every diagnostician, OCTA has great potential to show real-time blood flow in the retina so that doctors can identify the proper treatment earlier and more precisely.

Fluorescein Angiography

If your doctor thinks that you may have wet AMD, fluorescein angiography may be used to determine if there are abnormal blood vessels that are leaking below the macula. For this test, the doctor injects fluorescent dye into your arm and then traces its movement through the blood vessels in the retina. There, the appearance of fluorescent patches will show that the vessels are leaking. A special camera is used to take photos of the retina as the dye travels through the area.

STANDARD MEDICAL TREATMENT OPTIONS

Currently, there are no medical treatments for dry AMD, but there are "temporary" treatments for wet AMD. While they don't cure the disease, vision can return to near normal for a time or at least keep the individual functional for longer. These treatments are discussed below.

Treatments for macular degeneration have changed over the past several years. At one time, doctors used lasers in the treatment of the wet form of macular degeneration. A laser would burn or clot the tiny blood vessels that had grown near the macula to stop the flow of unwanted fluids. Unfortunately, that would leave a scar, and functional vision would be lost. However, recent developments in the treatment of AMD have taken different approaches to treating the wet form of the disease.

Photodynamic Therapy (PDT)

Approved by the FDA in 2000, *photodynamic therapy (PDT)* uses a light-sensitive medication called *verteporfin (Visudyne)* in combination with a laser light to eliminate leaking blood vessels. The medicine is injected into the bloodstream and collects in the abnormal blood vessels under the macula. The doctor then shines a low-intensity laser light into the eye, causing a chemical reaction that destroys the new blood vessels. This procedure does not restore function to damaged retinal cells, but by limiting the growth of abnormal blood vessels, it helps prevent further damage to the retina and further vision loss.

At one time, this was the primary treatment for wet AMD. Because it causes some scarring of the macula, it is now used only when more recently developed treatments prove to be ineffective.

Anti-VEGF Drugs

In 2004, it was discovered that a protein produced by the body called *vascular endothelial growth factor (VEGF)* stimulates the growth of the abnormal blood cells that cause retinal damage in the wet form of AMD. These findings led to the development of anti-VEGF drugs, which inhibit the actions of VEGF. Like photodynamic therapy, discussed above, these drugs do not cure AMD or restore the function of damaged cells, but they do help to preserve remaining vision.

The first anti-VEGF drug developed was *pegaptanib (Macugen)*. Pegaptanib works by blocking an essential signal that causes abnormal blood vessels to grow. The doctor injects pegaptanib into the back of the eye about every six weeks. Since there are no pain receptors in this area, the procedure involves only a bit of discomfort or pressure without any significant pain.

The second anti-VEGF drug developed is *ranibizumab (Lucentis)*. Like pegaptanib, it inhibits blood vessel growth, thereby protecting those cells that are still healthy. A third drug, called *bevacizumab* (Avastin)—which was originally used for metastatic colorectal cancer—is not FDA-approved for use on AMD, but is being used "off-label," and has been effective in halting the progression of AMD. A randomized controlled trial found that bevacizumab and ranibizumab had similar efficacy. Both generally yield better results than pegaptanib.

Another recent entry into the AMD market is *aflibercept (Eylea)*. Its action is similar to that of ranibizumab and bevacizumab, but since it has a slightly higher "receptivity" to the retina, it allows the retina to retain its function longer.

Combination Treatments

Some newer techniques involve using some of the above-mentioned drugs in combination. Your doctor can best evaluate your response to these medications and decide if combination therapy is warranted. Recent research has shown that the effectiveness of these treatments lessens with time and that by combining two drugs, a more positive result can be achieved.

Note that a number of considerations should be discussed with your doctor before you make the decision to begin therapy with a particular drug or drugs. First, be sure to review the side effects of these treatments. Anti-VEGF drugs can cause side effects such as increased eye pressure, vitreous bleeding, retinal tears or detachment, and macular hole. Since VEGF stimulates the growth of new blood vessels not just in the eye but also all over the body, when the action of this protein is inhibited, there may be systemic effects such as gastrointestinal perforations, hypertension, proteinuria, stroke, and myocardial infarction. The good news is that because the injections provide a low level of anti-VEGF serum, physical side effects are unlikely.

Another topic you will want to discuss with your doctor is cost, which varies from drug to drug. The cost of ranibizumab, for instance, is about forty-five times that of bevacizumab. Insurance companies do cover these treatments to some degree, but before beginning treatment, you should determine how much your particular policy will cover.

Nutritional Options

Currently, the only standard nutritional treatment recommended for age-related macular degeneration is the supplement formulation that was developed by the AGE-Related Eye Disease Study (AREDS). This study tested the effect on AMD of a specific set of nutrients, which did have a positive outcome in slowing the progression of

AMD. In Chapter 5, we will review that study and discuss how it applies to AMD.

It should be noted that AREDS supplementation has shown positive results only in mid- to late-stage AMD, and has succeeded only in slowing the progress of AMD, not in stopping the progress of AMD or reversing damage. Many doctors simply default to the AREDS formula because of the excellent design of the study. We, however, have looked at many other studies that use nutrients other than those in the AREDS formula, and have found that additional supplements can make a difference in the course of AMD. We will review these options in Chapters 6 and 7 and look at beneficial dietary changes in Part Three.

ALTERNATIVE TREATMENT OPTIONS

So far, we have discussed conventional medical treatment options for AMD. However, there are also alternative (non-standard) treatments that have shown some positive results. None of these treatments has received FDA approval to treat AMD, but since some encouraging results have been experienced, we want you to know a little more about each of these treatments. Also included is a look at cannabis—a substance that has not yet been tested as a treatment for AMD, but has properties that may make it a valuable ally in the war against macular degeneration.

Hyperbaric Oxygen Therapy

In *hyperbaric oxygen therapy (HBOT),* an individual breathes pure oxygen in a pressurized room or tube. This is a well-established treatment for decompression sickness and several other medical problems, and is FDA-approved for eye conditions such as central retinal artery occlusion and diabetic retinopathy. Researchers believe that it may be a potential treatment for AMD because a lack of oxygen is partly responsible for the macula's decline. Also, HBOT's supersaturated oxygen environment promotes eye cell regeneration and healing and also aids the body's production of stem cells, which can transform into the specialized cells that are involved in vision.

A few studies have investigated the use of HBOT in the treatment of AMD, where it can be effective in reactivating the "not-yet-dead" cells at the margins of the atrophic (functional loss) lesions and possibly stimulating the remaining retinal cells to a higher level of function. Significant improvements in visual acuity and field of vision have been observed after therapy. However, significant side effects can occur as well. These effects have included temporarily blurred vision caused by swelling of the lens and cornea, which usually resolves in two to four weeks. In addition, there have been reports that cataracts may progress following HBOT. A rare side effect has been blindness secondary to optic neuritis (inflammation of the optic nerve). The possible benefits of this treatment, however, outweigh the side effects, which do not occur often.

Acupuncture

A technique used in traditional Chinese medicine, *acupuncture* involves the insertion of extremely thin needles through the skin at specific points in the body for the purpose of balancing the flow of energy. Some acupuncture practitioners believe that this treatment can benefit people with AMD by stimulating blood flow to the eye. (Note that the needles are *not* inserted in the eye.) Research has shown that acupuncture does increase blood flow to the eye, so in theory, this seems plausible.

In Traditional Chinese Medicine (TCM) theory, AMD is due to blood deficiency and Qi (pronounced "chee") deficiency. In TCM, the liver is the blood-storing organ. Blood deficiency of the liver can lead to malnutrition of the eye. The therapeutic goal, then, is to replenish the liver and kidney and thereby increase circulation, and to resolve the presence of mucus and "dampness" that can block the circulation in the eyes.

It should be noted that although acupuncture is not an FDA-approved treatment for AMD, the American Medical Association does accept acupuncture techniques. The level of improvement is likely dependent on the stage of the disease and the length of time it has been developing.

Microcurrent Stimulation

Microcurrent stimulation uses low levels of electrical current to enhance circulation and cellular healing. In the case of AMD, by attaching small probes to the skin around the eye, practitioners apply electrical stimulation to nerve fibers with the goal of increasing circulation to the eye, stimulating the function of the retinal cells and reducing scar tissue. The technique is similar to that of transcutaneous electrical nerve stimulators (TENS), which have been used on other parts of the body with some success.

The use of microcurrent stimulation has shown positive results in the treatment of AMD. In a study published in *Clinical Ophthalmology*, twice as many patients treated with microcurrent stimulation showed a sizeable increase in visual acuity—which was measured before and after each treatment session—compared with those who experienced deterioration, and when deterioration did occur, it was very slight. In addition to providing benefits such as increased circulation, this therapy has been shown to boost the production of ATP, the major source of cellular energy. Since decreased levels of ATP are associated with AMD, an increase in ATP should be helpful for the person with macular degeneration.

The bottom line is that clinical studies have validated the effectiveness of using microcurrent stimulation to treat macular degeneration. Since this therapy can actually worsen vision if the settings on the microcurrent machines are wrong, it is essential to work with a practitioner who is experienced in using this therapy.

Cannabis (Marijuana)

While cannabis continues to be listed as a "Schedule 1" drug—that is, it is considered illegal and of no medical benefit by federal law— recent research has demonstrated that it can help heal the body. In fact, in 1999, the US Patent Office issued a patent for *cannabinoids* (the active chemical compounds in marijuana) to the National Institutes of Health, stating that cannabis is an effective antioxidant and nerve protection factor.

There are over one hundred cannabinoids in marijuana, and they have been found to relieve an array of symptoms. These substances activate receptor sites in the cells, and the eye area does have cannabinoid receptors. In a ground-breaking Finnish study, cannabis was found to lower eye pressure in glaucoma patients. While this doesn't specifically relate to AMD, it does show that cannabis can positively affect the eyes. Moreover, it is known that cannabidiol—one of the cannabinoids—has an anti-inflammatory effect on the retina. Cannibinoids have also been shown to inhibit the VEGF growth associated with wet macular degeneration.

At this point, no studies have been devoted to the treatment of AMD with cannabis. But considering the substances present in the plant, eventually, cannabinoid therapy may prove to be safe and effective for the millions of people suffering from macular degeneration.

CONCLUSION

Positive trends in the treatment of AMD continue to be established, and more medications currently are in the pipeline. However, at this time, neither form of macular degeneration—wet or dry—is medically or surgically curable by traditional medical treatments. Fortunately, as you will learn later in the book, there is much you can do to help prevent, slow, or even reverse AMD through nutritional supplementation and diet. In addition, as you will discover in the next chapter, while some risk factors for AMD cannot be changed—your genetics, for instance—other risk factors *can* be modified, providing you with better protection against macular degeneration.

3

What Are the Risk Factors for Macular Degeneration?

A s we age, there is a greater risk of getting a number of disorders, especially age-related macular degeneration. We do not know for sure who will or will not get the disease, but we do know the risk factors that can increase your chance of developing AMD. This chapter will discuss the various factors—environmental, genetic, and lifestyle-related—that have been shown to play a role in the development of macular degeneration. Although some of these factors, such as gender and age, cannot be modified, fortunately, some can. For instance, people who smoke can reduce their risk of developing this disorder by giving up tobacco. This is good news, because it means that you can take steps to delay or prevent the occurrence of AMD and possibly slow its progress if it has already begun.

THE RISK FACTORS

While we do not have a *definitive* list of causes for AMD, scientists have homed in on a number of factors that are shared by patients who get the disease. Some of these are genetic, but most are under our control. The following are the more common factors associated with macular degeneration.

■ AGE

This is obvious considering that the name of the disorder is *age-related* macular degeneration. AMD usually occurs in people over the age of fifty, and in the United States, it is the most common cause of vision loss in this age group. About 0.4 percent of people between ages fifty and sixty have the disease, while it occurs in 0.7 percent of people sixty to seventy, 2.3 percent of those seventy and eighty, and nearly 12 percent of people over eighty years old. As many as 1.6 million people in the United States have some form of age-related macular degeneration. With the aging of the population, this number is likely to double by 2050.

■ CORONARY HEART DISEASE

Coronary heart disease (CHD) is a condition in which a waxy substance called plaque builds up inside the arteries that deliver oxygen-rich blood to the heart muscle. Thus, an alternate name for this disorder is *coronary artery disease (CAD)*. The buildup of plaque reduces the flow of oxygen to the heart.

Studies have shown that there is a correlation between CHD and AMD. This is understandable, as CHD reduces the flow of blood not only to the heart, but also to other organs, including the eyes. As a result, vision can be greatly affected. Moreover, CHD and AMD may share similar risk factors and common mechanisms, such as the formation of plaque. This makes sense, since the drusen that form in the lining of the back of the retina are made up largely of calcium and cholesterol, which are also components of plaque. It's easy to see why CHD is a risk factor for macular degeneration.

■ GENDER

Gender also factors into the incidence of AMD. Women over the age of seventy-five have double the chance of developing AMD when compared with men of the same age. Low levels of estrogen in post-menopausal women may increase the risk for the condition. Although there is some suggestion that postmenopausal estrogen therapy may protect against AMD, more research needs to be conducted in this area to confirm these findings. Additionally, the disease is more likely to progress to a stage that causes severe vision loss in women because they have longer average life spans than men.

■ GENETICS AND EPIGENETICS

Some studies have shown that AMD may, in part, be inherited. This means that if you have one or more immediate relatives with AMD, you are at a higher risk for developing the condition. It is estimated that up to 70 percent of AMD risk is attributable to the more than fifteen genes that may contribute to this disease. A simple cheek-swab test can assess your likelihood of the disease advancing to a late stage.

Epigenetics is the study of the mechanisms that switch genes on and off, determining whether or not they get expressed. To put it another way, you can have a gene for AMD, but if factors like nutrition or the environment cause the gene to be dormant, AMD does not occur. If factors cause the gene to become active, however, AMD develops.

Epigenetics is a new area of study. We don't fully understand what causes genes to be turned on or off, and it is certainly beyond the scope of this book to review this fascinating and complex field. But we do know that by following a healthful lifestyle, you can make it more likely that your good genes will be expressed and your bad genes will remain dormant.

■ HYPERTENSION

The eyes provide the perfect way to view the blood vessels without using an invasive procedure. In fact, this is the only place in the body where the small blood vessels can be seen clearly. One of the most prominent features is the pattern of blood vessels that line the inside of the eye, lying on top of the retina (when viewed by looking through the pupil). By examining this area, doctors can look for the damage associated with high blood pressure (hypertension), including thickened, narrowed, or burst blood vessels. This damage can lead to bleeding in the eye, the death of nerve cells, and other problems that can cause vision loss. It's not surprising, then, that several studies have shown a correlation between patients with hypertension and the onset of AMD. (To learn more about hypertension and its effect on the body, see page 44 of Chapter 4.)

■ INACTIVITY

We often hear how important exercise is for every aspect of our health. Our eyes, too, can benefit from regular exercise and activity.

One study monitored 4,000 people age forty-three to eighty-six for fifteen years. After considering a number of risk factors, such as age, it was found that people who lead an active lifestyle were 70-percent less likely to develop AMD during the follow-up period. In this case, those considered to have an "active lifestyle" walked at least two miles a day, three times a week. Other studies, too, have found connections between regular exercise and a reduced risk of eye ailments such as wet age-related macular degeneration.

One explanation for these study results may be that, as you have already learned, AMD is associated with high blood pressure and coronary heart disease. Regular exercise—along with a healthy diet—is key to eliminating these two risk factors. (You will learn more about exercise in Chapter 12.)

■ LIGHT EXPOSURE

The light that enters the eye is composed of many "wavelengths." You are probably familiar with some of them, such as ultraviolet light. The cornea and lens of the eye absorb most of the ultraviolet light, but they allow the blue light—the highest-energy visible light—to reach the retina, and laboratory studies have shown that too much exposure to blue light can damage the light-sensitive cells in delicate retinal tissue. A paper published by the American Medical Association reported that the blue rays of the light spectrum appear to hasten the progress of AMD more than other rays in the spectrum. This is an area of study that has yet to be firmly established, since AMD can occur in populations where excessive blue light is not prevalent.

Many eye-care providers are concerned about blue light exposure that results from the use of computer screens, smart phones, and other digital devices. But the amount of blue light emitted by digital devices is minimal, and the jury is still out on these devices' contribution to AMD. It's important to remember, however, that the sun contains *all* of the wavelengths of light, and that cellular damage from the sun can, over time, lead to deterioration of the macula. To minimize damage from the sun, experts recommend wearing sunglasses that reduce exposure to harmful rays through UV and blue light protection. (To learn more about protecting your eyes from light exposure, see page 211 of Chapter 12.)

■ OBESITY AND A POOR DIET

Over sixty studies link excess weight to eye disease in general, and many of them link obesity to AMD in particular. Most likely, this is true for several reasons.

As you know, excess body weight predisposes people to disorders such as coronary heart disease and hypertension, both of which are associated with AMD. Macular degeneration is directly related to the vascular system, and excess weight is known to create problems that lead to the deterioration of blood vessels in the eye.

The macula's fragile cells are also highly susceptible to damage from the molecules called *free radicals*—atoms with unpaired electrons that form in the body when oxygen interacts with certain molecules. The body fights free radicals with antioxidants, but a low intake of antioxidants due to a poor diet can leave the body open to the free radicals' harmful actions. Additionally, alcohol may deplete the body of antioxidants. An excessive intake of saturated fats and cholesterol—two substances that are characteristic of poor diets—is also involved in producing free-radical reactions, so these substances can lead to AMD in several ways. (Note that you'll learn more about diet in Chapters 8 through 11. To learn more about obesity, see page 40 of Chapter 4.)

■ DIABETES AND PREDIABETES

Diabetes—an abnormal metabolism of carbohydrates that leads to elevated blood glucose levels—is also one of the top causes of blindness in the United States today. Typically, diabetes weakens blood vessel walls, causing the small blood vessels inside the eye to become more fragile. When this happens, fluids and blood leak into the center of the eye. There, the blood eventually clots and pulls the retina away from the inside of the eye, and vision is lost. This condition is known as *diabetic retinopathy*. Recent studies suggest that the swelling of the macula due to diabetes, diabetic retinopathy, and AMD are similar in that they are all conditions characterized by a breakdown of the blood-retinal barrier, inflammatory processes, and a weakness in the integrity of the blood vessels in the eye.

In prediabetes, blood glucose levels are higher than normal, but not high enough for a diagnosis of fully developed diabetes. Lifestyle changes at important at this point because people with prediabetes are very likely to progress to type 2 diabetes. Your doctor will let you know if you have prediabetes, and he will assess whether any long-term damage—including damage to the eyes—has already occurred. (To learn more about prediabetes and diabetes, see page 46 of Chapter 4.)

■ RACE

There is a clear association between age-related macular degeneration and race, with some groups being more likely to develop the disease than others. The incidence of early and late AMD is highest in Caucasians (5.3 percent), intermediate in Asians (4.5 percent) and Hispanics (3.3 percent), and lowest in African Americans, who have a 70-percent lower risk of developing early AMD than Caucasians. While researchers haven't been able to pinpoint the cause of these differences, one consideration is the higher amount of overall pigment in the eyes of African Americans, which can reduce the amount of high-intensity light that reaches the retina. This theory appears to be borne out by the fact that in Caucasian patients, AMD is significantly more common in individuals with blue or hazel irises than in those with brown irises.

■ SMOKING

Studies have shown that smokers are from two to five times more likely than nonsmokers to develop age-related macular degeneration. The more people smoke and the longer they smoke, the higher the risk of the disease.

Researchers have offered a number of explanations for this increased risk. Smoking appears to speed the deterioration of macular cells by interfering with the action of protective nutrients such as lutein and zeaxanthin. It also increases the number of damaging free radicals in the bloodstream. Smoking has been shown to narrow the blood vessels, reducing the flow of blood and oxygen to the eye. It may even reduce the density of the macular pigment, which protects the eye from oxidative damage.

Both current smokers and past smokers have an increased risk of developing macular degeneration, but quitting can make a positive difference. Former smokers have only a slightly increased risk of developing AMD when compared with people who have never smoked. (To learn more about the effects of smoking, see page 209 of Chapter 12.)

■ METABOLIC SYNDROME

Metabolic syndrome is a cluster of disorders that include abdominal obesity, high triglycerides, low HDL ("good") cholesterol, high blood pressure, and high blood sugar levels. Since you are now aware that obesity, hypertension, and diabetes are all risk factors for AMD, it should make sense that when these disorders occur together, the risk for late AMD is greater. Chapter 4 focuses on metabolic syndrome—what it is and how it can be controlled.

CONCLUSION

You now know about a number of factors that can increase your risk for developing age-related macular degeneration. As we said at the start of this chapter, you can't do anything about some of these factors, but the majority of risk factors *can* be changed. To reduce the risk of damage to your macula, you can quit smoking if you now smoke; wear quality sunglasses with UV and blue light protection when you go outdoors; modify your diet to favor a healthy weight, lower blood pressure, and a lower risk of heart disease; and add physical activity to your daily life. If this seems like a tall order, don't worry; we've got you covered. In Parts Two and Three, you will learn what you need to know to improve what you eat and add eye-healthy nutrients to your diet. In Part Four, you will learn how to make critical lifestyle changes that can help maintain clear vision for as long as possible. But before we move onto the important actions you can take to safeguard your eyes, it's important to learn more about the last risk factor mentioned in this chapter—metabolic syndrome—which is the subject of the next chapter.

4

Metabolic Syndrome

In Chapter 3, you learned the risk factors for age-related macular degeneration, and the last one mentioned was metabolic syndrome (MetS). While you might have heard of this syndrome, you might not have a clear idea of what it is. This is understandable because metabolic syndrome—or Syndrome X, as it is sometimes called—doesn't have a neat, concise definition. Instead, it is a cluster of five conditions or risk factors that have been found to increase the incidence of cardiovascular disease and diabetes. Moreover, if you have just three of the five risk factors, you are considered to have MetS.

Over the years, metabolic syndrome has become exceedingly common—an epidemic, really—centered in the United States and the Western world. In one United States study, researchers analyzed data on almost 9,000 men and women of twenty years of age and older. In those adults ages sixty and above, about *40 percent* met the criteria for MetS. The frequency of this disorder increases with age. Considering its high incidence and its relationship to AMD, it makes sense to better understand this health issue.

This chapter examines each of the five risk factors for metabolic syndrome, explaining what they are and what they mean to your health in general and your eye health in particular. Just as important, it looks at what you can do to avoid or reverse MetS.

METABOLIC SYNDROME RISK FACTORS

As explained above, metabolic syndrome is a constellation of five risk factors. You need to have only three of the following health problems for your doctor to make the diagnosis of metabolic syndrome. As you read about these conditions, keep in mind that if any *one* of these risk factors becomes more severe, it increases your likelihood of developing macular degeneration.

Abdominal Obesity and Overall Obesity

Abdominal obesity is the first component of metabolic syndrome. This condition can be defined as a waist circumference that is greater than 40 inches in men and greater than 35 inches in women. People with abdominal obesity have an "apple" shape, with the extra pounds being found around the waist, rather than a "pear" shape, in which the extra pounds are found around the hips.

Although the size of your waist and the shape of your body can indicate whether you have abdominal obesity, you can more accurately determine this condition by calculating your waist-to-hip ratio. First, with your abdomen relaxed, measure around your waist at its narrowest point. Next, measure around your hips at their widest point, which is usually at the bony prominences. Then simply divide your waist circumference (in centimeters or inches) by your hip circumference. For example, a person with a 30-inch waist and 38-inch hips has a waist-to-hip ratio of approximately 0.79. (30 ÷ 38 = 0.789) According to the World Health Organization, the target ratio for men is less than .9, and the target ratio for women is less than .85. Anything above these ratios is considered abdominal obesity.

In addition to being a risk factor for metabolic syndrome, abdominal obesity has been linked directly to macular degeneration. According to research published by the University of Melbourne in Australia, patients who lower their waist-to-hip ratio decrease their risk of developing AMD. Why is abdominal fat linked to both metabolic syndrome and AMD? To put it simply, scientists have found that fat which accumulates in this region of the body is actually different from fat in other portions of the body. Excess belly fat makes insulin less able to control blood sugar, makes you eat more and store fat more easily, raises blood cholesterol levels, and raises blood pressure. It's no wonder that abdominal obesity is a risk factor for a number of disorders.

If you've read the previous chapter, you know that overall obesity is also a risk factor for AMD. When we talk about overall obesity, we mean that an individual has too much body fat, but that the fat is not concentrated in one area, as it is with abdominal obesity. When someone is obese, their risk of progression to late AMD is 32-percent higher than the risk of thinner individuals. Moreover, the greater the weight, the higher the risk for late AMD. One reason for this increased risk may be that people with higher body fat levels have been found to have less of the protective pigments lutein and zeaxanthin in the macula. Because both lutein and zeaxanthin are fat-soluble, they are easily stored in the fat tissue beneath the skin. When fat levels are normal, these compounds are more easily transported to the eye to help protect the retina in general, and the macula in particular. When fat levels are higher, transportation is more difficult, and the macula suffers. Of course, excess weight also increases the risk for other age-related diseases. For instance, someone with normal weight has a 4-percent risk of developing diabetes, while someone who is obese has a 25-percent risk. The risk for high blood pressure jumps from 16 percent to as much as 50 percent as you move from normal weight to obesity. Both of these disorders are associated with a higher incidence of AMD.

Doctors use a standard of measurement called the *body mass index (BMI)* to determine whether an individual is underweight, normal weight, overweight, or obese. Basically, the BMI compares an individual's weight and height by using the following formula:

$$BMI = \frac{\text{weight in pounds} \times 703}{\text{height in inches}^2}$$

If this is more math than you want to do, simply use one of the many BMI calculators that are available online, like those on the website of the Centers for Disease Control (CDC) or the USDA. (See pages 247 and 248 of the Resources list for contact information.) Normal weight is considered a BMI of 18.5 to 24.9, overweight is 25.0 to 29.9, and obesity is 30.0 and above. In a study based on data collected by the National Institutes of Health from 2011 to 2012, almost 40 percent of American men and 30 percent of American women were over-weight, and 35 percent of men and 37 percent of women were obese. These are staggering numbers.

This book is not intended to be a weight-loss guide. However, we know that by changing from the typical American diet to the Anti-AMD Diet, you can avoid both abdominal obesity and overall obesity. (See Chapters 8 to 11 for details.) Add some daily exercise (see pages 206 to 209), and there will be a "new" you—thinner and healthier, with a lower risk for AMD and a slew of other age-re-lated diseases.

High Triglycerides

Triglycerides are a type of fat found in your blood, so called because they are composed of three fatty acids attached to a chemical back-bone of glycerol. When you eat, any calories that aren't needed by the body for energy are converted into triglycerides and stored in your fat cells. They are later released for energy between meals. In fact, they are the primary source of energy for the body. But if you regularly eat more calories than you burn, you may have high triglycerides, or *hypertriglyceridemia.* Certain foods contain tri-glycerides, as well. While these substances are found in both animal and plant fats, trans fats and animal fats tend to elevate levels of tri-glycerides more than healthy fats. Sugar and alcohol can also raise triglyceride levels.

You doctor may have already measured this substance in your blood as part of a blood analysis called a *lipid profile* or *lipid panel,* which tests for total cholesterol, LDL ("bad") cholesterol, HDL ("good") cholesterol, and triglycerides. (You'll learn more about cho-lesterol on page 43.) Triglycerides less than 150 mg/dL are considered normal, 150 to 199 mg/dL are borderline high, 200 to 499 mg/dL are high, and 500 mg/dL or above are very high. High or borderline high triglycerides are a risk factor for metabolic syndrome, which increases your risk for heart disease and stroke.

The jury is still out on the connection between high triglycerides and AMD. While some studies have reported that high triglycerides are a risk factor for AMD, other studies have offered conflicting results. But since high triglycerides increase your risk for metabolic syndrome—which is a risk factor for not only cardiovascular disease but also macular degeneration—it is prudent to keep this substance within normal ranges.

There are many steps you can take to normalize high triglycerides. By switching to the Anti-AMD Diet, you will avoid some high-triglyceride food sources and also lose some weight. Just losing ten to twenty pounds can reduce your triglycerides by about 20 percent. Then add some aerobic exercise—the kind that increases your heart rate.

Your doctor may also want you to take nutritional supplements, including omega-3 fatty acids and/or niacin. The prescription drug Lovaza (omega-3-acid ethyl esters), which contains about 900 mg EPA and DHA, can reduce your triglycerides by 20 to 50 percent, and should be covered by health insurance. Off-the-shelf fish oil is another option, but be sure that the EPA and DHA levels add up to at least 900 mg. Another nutritional supplement that your doctor may prescribe is nicotinic acid or niacin, one of the B vitamins. Available by prescription as Niaspan Extended Release (niacin), it can lower your triglycerides by 20 to 50 percent, decrease your LDL ("bad") cholesterol by 5 to 25 percent, and increase your HDL ("good") cholesterol by 15 to 35 percent. But it can also have side effects, so discuss this medication with your doctor before beginning treatment.

Low High-Density Lipoprotein (HDL) Cholesterol

The third component of metabolic syndrome is low levels of high-density lipoprotein (HDL) cholesterol, or "good" cholesterol. HDL cholesterol is considered "good" because it helps remove cholesterol from your arteries. It's like a vacuum cleaner, sucking up extra cholesterol that is accumulating as plaque and taking it to your liver for safe disposal. By way of contrast, LDL cholesterol—low-density lipoprotein cholesterol—is considered "bad" because it contributes to fatty buildup in the arteries.

Like triglyceride levels, HDL cholesterol levels are usually determined by your doctor through a lipid panel or lipid profile. When it comes to HDL cholesterol, a higher number means a lower risk of health disorders. If your HDL score is greater than 60 mg/dL, that's good! For women, less than 50 mg/dl is too low; for men, less than 40 mg/dL is too low.

High levels of HDL cholesterol are protective against heart disease, and low levels of this substance increase the risk of heart disease and, of course, of metabolic syndrome. Is there a link between HDL cholesterol and macular degeneration? Strangely, some studies indicate that elevated HDL—which is normally considered good— are associated with a *higher* risk for AMD. Researchers are unsure of the cause of this finding. Does it mean, for instance, that patients with AMD have special problems with their HDL? Whatever the reason, because high HDL cholesterol is associated with greater cardiovascular health, it is prudent to do what you can to maintain high levels of this important substance.

If your HDL levels are too low, following the Anti-AMD Diet can help elevate them. (See Chapters 8 to 11.) Be sure to include olive oil and foods high in omega-3 fatty acids, such as salmon and sardines, in your meals. On days that you don't include these foods, take a fish oil supplement. Moderate alcohol intake may be helpful, but if you don't drink, don't start just to increase your HDL. If you smoke, take steps to stop the habit, and try to perform aerobic exercises for thirty minutes a day.

High Blood Pressure

High blood pressure (HBP), or hypertension, is another component of metabolic syndrome. *Blood pressure* is the force of blood pushing against the artery walls as the blood moves from the heart to all the organs. In *hypertension,* the blood places higher-than-normal force against artery walls as it moves through the body. There are no symptoms of this disorder, so you can walk around with it for years and have no clue as to the damage it is doing. The only way you can determine if you have hypertension is to have your healthcare provider take your blood pressure or to take it yourself with one of the many easy-to-use devices now available in drugstores.

Each blood pressure reading is made up of two numbers. The top number, or *systolic pressure*, measures the pressure in the arteries at the peak of a heartbeat, when the heart muscle contracts. The bottom number, or *diastolic pressure*, measures the pressure in the arteries between the heartbeats, when the heart muscle is relaxing. Therefore, the reading 130/90 mmHg (millimeters of mercury) indicates a systolic pressure of 130 and a diastolic pressure of 90. Here's what the readings mean:

- *Normal BP:* less than 120 systolic and less than 80 diastolic

- *Prehypertension:* 120 to 139 systolic or 81 to 89 diastolic

- *Hypertension:* 140 or more systolic or 90 or more diastolic

The leading cause of heart disease worldwide, hypertension affects 72 million Americans. When uncontrolled, high blood pressure damages and weakens the blood vessels. Artery walls can become less elastic, limiting blood flow; and blood vessels can narrow, rupture, or leak. High blood pressure can also cause blood clots to form, blocking blood flow. Over time, this damage can lead to heart attack; stroke; or *aneurysm*—a weakening of an artery wall. And hypertension can harm much more than the heart. Blood vessels are injured all over the body, including the brain, which can lead to mini-strokes, major strokes, dementia, and reduced cognitive abilities. Untreated, HBP also damages the micro-vessels that carry oxygen and nutrients to the eyes and carry away waste products. This can lead to deterioration of the retina and loss of vision. It can also cause blood vessels located under the retina to leak, resulting in fluid buildup, scarring, and distorted vision. By killing off nerve cells and causing bleeding, hypertension can even damage the optic nerve, which carries visual messages to the brain. It's easy to understand why hypertension is associated with so many health disorders, including AMD.

Because high blood pressure can cause so many problems, if you have prehypertension or hypertension, you will want to do everything you can to lower your blood pressure. Start by following the

Anti-AMD Diet. (See Chapters 8 to 11 for details.) Be sure to include generous amounts of fruits and vegetables, nuts, seeds, beans, whole grains, and cold water fish, as this will provide blood pressure-lowering nutrients. Your doctor may prescribe the DASH Diet—Dietary Approaches to Stop Hypertension—which is similar to the Anti-AMD Diet. Either diet would be a good choice, and either one can help you lose weight, which can play a major role in lowering blood pressure. In fact, losing just ten pounds can make an important difference in your BP. Remember, too, to lower your salt intake.

You'll also want to quit smoking and start exercising, both of which can help to lower your blood pressure. (You'll learn more about these healthy lifestyle choices in Chapter 12.). If you feel stressed, it's important to find ways to relax. Exercise can be a big part of that, but you also might want to look into yoga and specific relaxation techniques.

Certain supplements can also help you lower your blood pressure. Below, you'll find a few that have been found to be particularly effective. They may help you avoid taking medication for hypertension, or, if you are already on medication, they may enable you to lower your dose. Any changes in dosage, however, should be made only in consultation with your physician.

- *Magnesium.* Take 400 mg every day.

- *Garlic.* Take 500 to 1,000 mg per day.

- *Coenzyme Q$_{10}$.* Take 200 to 300 mg per day.

- *Fish oil (omega-3 fatty acids).* Take about 1,000 mg total EPA and DHA (check back label).

Elevated Fasting Blood Glucose

When you eat a food containing carbohydrates, the body breaks the carbs down into sugar, or glucose, which then enters the bloodstream. As blood glucose levels rise, the pancreas produces the hormone insulin, which tells the cells to absorb the glucose for immediate use as energy or for storage. As the cells absorb the glucose, the blood levels of glucose fall.

Blood glucose levels vary throughout the day. Following are normal levels:

- Upon waking, blood glucose should be under 100 mg/dL. (This is referred to as a fasting blood glucose level.)

- Before a meal, blood glucose should be between 70 and 99 mg/dL.

- Two hours after a meal, blood glucose should be less than 140 mg/dL.

An individual is said to have *prediabetes* when the fasting blood glucose level is 100 mg/dL or higher. At this point, the blood sugar level is considered a risk factor for metabolic syndrome. When blood sugar is 126 mg/dL or higher on two separate tests, a diagnosis of *diabetes* is made.

Persistently high blood sugar causes damage throughout the body. By injuring the nerves, it can decrease or block the movement of nerve impulses through the arms, legs, organs, and other parts of the body. Nerve damage can also lead to hearing loss and even Alzheimer's disease.

By harming large blood vessels, high blood sugar can damage the heart, brain, and legs. People with diabetes are more likely to have a heart attack or a stroke.

High blood sugar also causes damage to the tiny blood vessels throughout the body, especially in the feet, kidneys, and eyes. People with diabetes may experience burning, tingling, or even numbness in their feet. Since loss of sensation makes individuals more susceptible to injury, this can lead to infection in the feet and toes. Kidney damage is another common result of persistently high blood sugar. And, of course, high blood sugar can damage the small blood vessels in the retina, leading to eye disease, including AMD.

Considering all the problems that can be caused by high blood sugar, it's important to do all you can to normalize your glucose levels if they are now elevated. Of course, you should closely follow the Anti-AMD Diet. (See Chapters 8 to 11.) Fruits, vegetables, whole grain cereals, nuts, beans, seeds, low-fat milk products, lean protein, and cold water fish can help maintain normal blood sugar levels and offer protection against complications. Fiber is especially important, as it can improve glucose levels by slowing the absorption of sugar. The Anti-AMD Diet can also help you lose weight, which will greatly improve your blood sugar numbers. Be sure to exercise, too—at least thirty minutes a day, even if you just go for a long walk. (See Chapter 12.) This is another way to control your weight and keep your blood glucose in the healthy range.

Certain supplements have shown value in managing blood glucose levels. The following four have proven especially helpful. If your doctor has placed you on medication to treat your condition, be sure to discuss these supplements with him before taking them.

- *Magnesium.* Take 400 mg every day.

Risk Factors for Prediabetes and Diabetes

Researchers don't completely understand why some people develop prediabetes and diabetes, and others do not. However, the following risk factors increase the chance that an individual will develop these conditions:

- **Weight.** The more fatty tissue you have, the more resistant your cells are to insulin—which means that glucose will remain in the bloodstream rather than being used by your cells.

- **Inactivity.** The less active you are, the greater your risk, because physical activity is needed to use up glucose to fuel the body.

- **Family history.** If diabetes runs in your family—if a parent or sibling has type 2 diabetes—your risk is higher.

- **Race.** African Americans, Hispanics, American Indians, and Asian Americans are at higher risk for diabetes than Caucasians.

- **Age.** As you get older, your risk for diabetes increases. However, this may be due to inactivity and increasing weight.

- **Gestational diabetes.** If you developed gestational diabetes during pregnancy, your risk of developing diabetes is higher.

- *Chromium picolinate.* Take 1,000 mcg in two doses (500 mcg each) every day.

- *Cinnamon.* Take 1 to 6 g every day. (Start with 1 g, and increase as needed.)

- *L-carnitine.* Take 2 g or less per day.

METABOLIC SYNDROME AND AMD

Clearly, metabolic syndrome is a risk factor for AMD. This should not be a surprise, since in Chapter 3, you learned that obesity, hypertension, and diabetes are each risk factors for AMD. In addition, studies

- **Polycystic ovary syndrome.** If you have been diagnosed with polycystic ovary syndrome, your risk of developing diabetes is higher.

- **High blood pressure.** If you have blood pressure over 140/90 mmHg, you have a greater risk of developing diabetes.

- **Abnormal cholesterol and triglyceride levels.** If you have elevated triglyceride levels and low levels of HDL cholesterol—the "good" cholesterol—your risk of developing diabetes is higher.

Although it is not listed as an "official" risk factor, studies show that a high consumption of sugar-sweetened beverages, artificially sweetened beverages, and fruit juice—apart from increasing body weight—are significantly associated with getting diabetes. In global studies, researchers reported that diabetes is 20-percent higher in countries with a high availability of high-fructose corn syrup compared with countries with low availability. Scientists at the University of Colorado said, "The intake of added sugars, such as from table sugar (sucrose) and high-fructose corn syrup, has increased dramatically in the last hundred years and correlates closely with the rise in obesity, metabolic syndrome, and diabetes." Fortunately, you can avoid sweetened beverages and many of the other risk factors listed above, substantially decreasing your risk for both prediabetes and diabetes—as well as for AMD.

have shown a link between metabolic syndrome and macular degeneration. The Blue Mountains Eye Study in Australia was specifically designed to investigate the relationship between metabolic syndrome and its components with early and late age-related macular degeneration. Over a ten-year period, a group of more than 2,200 individuals age forty-nine and older were followed, and standard retinal images were used to track the development of AMD. The study showed that MetS was connected with the incidence of late AMD. Of the five components of metabolic syndrome, obesity, high glucose, and high triglycerides were associated with the eye disease. There was no evidence that MetS and its components affected the risk of early AMD.

CONCLUSION

If you have been diagnosed with metabolic syndrome, consider it an urgent wake-up call. Remember that MetS is not a disease in itself but a group of symptoms that can predict future more serious conditions, including heart disease, diabetes, and age-related macular degeneration. It's time to drastically improve your eating habits with the Anti-AMD Diet, to lower your weight, and to exercise daily. You have the power to avoid or eliminate abdominal obesity, high triglycerides, low HDL cholesterol, high blood pressure, and elevated blood glucose—all of the risk factors for metabolic syndrome. In the chapters that follow, you will learn about the many steps you can take to improve your overall health, reverse the course of MetS, and prevent or halt the progression of age-related macular degeneration.

Part Two

Macular Degeneration and Supplements

5

$\mathscr{T}$he AREDS Trials

N ow that we have reviewed the disease process of AMD and learned about the risk factors for this disorder, we are ready to look at what you can do to stop or at least slow the progression of the disease. As you learned in Chapter 2, the medications now available to treat AMD address only the later stages of the wet form of the condition. Fortunately, you can positively affect the course of AMD earlier in the process through other forms of treatment.

A number of years ago, researchers set out to investigate whether macular disease can be prevented or treated through the use of *micronutrients:* nutrients (such as vitamins and minerals) that are required by the body in minute amounts. The studies they conducted—the Age-Related Eye Disease Studies, or AREDS—established gold-standard clinical evidence that specific supplements help protect the eyes from AMD. The nutritional approach based on the AREDS formula is now the most widely accepted means of combating this disorder. This chapter looks at these important studies and at the nutrients that were found to be crucial to eye health.

THE AREDS STUDIES

During the last two decades, several studies have shown the benefits of nutritional supplements for patients with age-related macular degeneration. Of these studies, the two AREDS trials have had the greatest impact on clinical eye care.

The First AREDS Trial

The initial Age-Related Eye Disease Study was the first large-scale clinical trial designed to evaluate the effectiveness of high-dose levels of antioxidants and mineral supplements on age-related macular degeneration and cataracts. According to the study's documents, AREDS was undertaken largely because of the widespread public use of certain vitamins and minerals to treat these two eye conditions and the absence of definitive studies on the safety and efficacy of their use. However, some authorities believe that the formulators developed this study to show that vitamins and minerals were *not* effective in changing the course of AMD and cataracts.

The National Eye Institute (NEI), part of the National Institutes of Health, sponsored AREDS. It proposed the concept for AREDS in 1986, and developed the protocol and supplement formula between 1990 and 1992. The first participants enrolled in November 1992, and recruitment was complete in three years, with the final participants (numbering about 3,640) enrolled in July 1996. The stages of disease ranged from no evidence of AMD in either eye, to advanced AMD with vision loss in one eye, but good vision (at least 20/30) in the other eye. Of the participants, 56 percent were female, and the median age was sixty-nine. About 90 percent of all participants were followed for a minimum of five years; about 2 percent were lost to follow-up; about 1 percent were in the study for less than five years; and about 7 percent died before five years. About half of the participants were given the nutrient formulation, and half were given a placebo that contained no nutrients. Before the trial and at each successive checkup, each participant was tested to measure both visual acuity and the size of the drusen—the yellow deposits behind the retina that can indicate macular degeneration.

The nutrients used in the study were selected on the basis of both the public's extensive use of certain supplements to treat AMD and cataracts, and the products' commercial availability. They included:

- Beta-carotene (15 mg)
- Zinc (80 mg)
- Vitamin C (500 mg)
- Copper (2 mg)
- Vitamin E (400 IU)

The Results of the First AREDS Trial

The results of the first AREDS study were both important and encouraging. Those participants who took the AREDS formula experienced a slowing of the progression of the disease from the intermediate to late stages. The study did *not* show any effect on the start, reversal, or halting of the disease at any stage. The AREDS formula also had no statistically significant effects on the progression of cataracts.

People who had previously doubted the power of nutritional supplementation on AMD were surprised by the results, and the eye-care community began reconsidering the role of nutrients in the course of the disease. Unfortunately, this led some doctors to prescribe the AREDS formula not only for people in the intermediate to late stages of the disorder, but also to people with early AMD—a group that had not responded to the formula during the trial. Nevertheless, a positive step had been taken in AMD research when AREDS successfully demonstrated that nutrition could affect the course of macular degeneration.

The Second AREDS Trial

In 2002, the NEI initiated a second study called AREDS2, which used a modified nutritional formula. While the original AREDS study had not shown any significant effect on cataract progression, because this second study adjusted the nutrients, researchers felt that this mode of treatment warranted another look. As far as treatment for AMD, researchers wanted to see if they could improve upon the results of the original AREDS formula and also enhance patient safety.

A similar number of study participants—4,200 subjects—were included in AREDS2, but there were several differences in the types of participants chosen. Because the AREDS1 formulation had not proven effective in preventing AMD or helping people with early AMD, all of the participants in AREDS2 had intermediate AMD in both eyes or advanced AMD in one eye. AREDS2 also included an older population; more diabetics; and, according to dietary questionnaires filled out by the participants, people who were better nourished. Perhaps most important, this study did not have a placebo group. Because the original formula had shown a positive result, for ethical reasons, the control group in AREDS2 received the nutrients used in the first study rather than a placebo.

Along with the original AREDS formula, the new test formula included three more commercially available nutrients: lutein (10 mg), zeaxanthin (2 mg), and fish oil (1,000 mg). Different sub-groups of participants used slightly different combinations of nutrients. In one subgroup, no beta-carotene was included because research from other studies had indicated that high levels of beta-carotene could increase the risk of lung cancer in smokers and former smokers. Another subgroup used a lower level of zinc (25 mg rather than the original 80 mg). Because of the variety of formulas used, the trial resulted in a flurry of statistics that had to be interpreted.

The Results of AREDS2

Research studies are guided by statistics, and as you may know, there are raw statistics and there are "adjusted" statistics. This means that the results of any study can be presented in a way that supports a certain point of view. It is not our intention to prove or disprove the conclusions of the AREDS trials, but we do want to look at these trials with a critical eye so that we can better evaluate the stated results.

The primary analysis of AREDS2 showed that this new formula was no better than the original formula. A *primary analysis* is the original analysis of data in a research study. It is what one typically imagines as the application of statistical methods. A *secondary analysis* is a re-analysis of data for the purpose of answering the original research question, or answering new questions with old data. Some studies have *tertiary*, or third-level, analyses. We have to realize that in this AREDS2 study, the "placebo"—the original AREDS formula—reduced the progression of intermediate AMD to advanced AMD by 25 percent. Thus, the AREDS2 analysis had to determine if the new formula could achieve an *additional* reduction.

Although the initial analysis was disappointing, once the statisticians dug a little deeper into the numbers (in their tertiary analysis) and adjusted for the effects of the original formula, they found that the AREDS2 formula had significantly slowed the progression of the disease. Although the researchers had anticipated an additional reduction of 25 percent, the added reduction of 19 percent was significant. Just like the original study, there was little effect on the progression of cataracts.

Patients who, according to their dietary questionnaires, had the lowest dietary intake of lutein and zeaxanthin showed a further reduction of progression toward advanced AMD when taking these supplements as part of the AREDS2 formula. The investigators found no significant changes in the effectiveness of the formulation when they removed beta-carotene or lowered zinc. This was an important conclusion, because the beta-carotene in the original AREDS formula was known to place smokers and former smokers at a higher risk for lung cancer. Omega-3 supplementation via fish oil did not result in a significant reduction in the progression of AMD, but as you'll learn later in the book, omega-3s have shown positive results in later studies.

Based on AREDS2, the newly designed formula now includes:

- Vitamin C (500 mg)
- Copper (2 mg)
- Vitamin E (400 IU)
- Lutein (10 mg)
- Zinc (80 mg)
- Zeaxanthin (2 mg)

People often ask if you can achieve this high level of nutrient intake through food alone. That would be nearly impossible. However, previous studies have suggested that people who have diets rich in green, leafy vegetables—a good source of lutein and zeaxanthin—have a lower risk of developing AMD. As already mentioned, in the AREDS2 trial, those subjects who seemed to benefit most from taking lutein and zeaxanthin were those who received little of these nutrients in their diet. These participants had a 26-percent reduced risk of developing advanced AMD compared with those who did not receive the supplements. This result seems to emphasize the fact that while nutritional supplementation is important, diet and lifestyle can also make a crucial difference in the progression of the disease. We will review these concepts in detail in Parts Three and Four.

Problems with the AREDS Studies

The AREDS and AREDS2 studies are generally recognized as gold standard studies because they are the only randomized controlled trials (RCTs) supported by the National Eye Institute for age-related macular degeneration. When we say that AREDS is a *randomized controlled trial*, we mean that the subjects are assigned to different groups at random (by chance), and there is a standard of comparison, or a control. While both AREDS formulas did show some positive results, recall that they did not show any effect on the starting, halting, or reversing of AMD. They simply slowed down the progression of the disease from the intermediate to late stage. Moreover, these formulas are limited considering that many other studies point to additional nutrients that support eye health in many other ways. We will review some of those studies below and discuss further nutritional supplements in the next few chapters.

To Zinc or Not to Zinc

One of the most controversial aspects of the AREDS and AREDS2 studies relates to the amount of zinc used. The mineral zinc plays a role in hundreds of chemical processes in the body. But as with all nutrients, more is not necessarily better. Zinc was included in this formula because studies in the early 1980s showed that it benefits eye function by transporting vitamin A into the retina. The AREDS study was designed to assess whether zinc, alone or in combination with the vitamin/antioxidant formulation, could slow the progression of AMD. Formulations that included zinc also had copper added to offset potential zinc-induced copper-deficiency anemia. Zinc competes with copper for absorption in the human body, and the use of zinc supplements can cause an imbalance of these minerals.

The National Academy of Medicine (NAM) makes recommendations on the essential nutrients needed for health and fitness. The

Recommended Daily Intake (RDI) of zinc is 15 mg per day for the average adult. The maximum recommendation for an adult is 40 mg. However, the amount used in the AREDS study was *twice* that, at 80 mg. Side effects of zinc when taken in large doses have included diarrhea, abdominal cramps, and vomiting, which usually occur within three to ten hours of dosing. AREDS2 tested both 80 mg and 25 mg and found no difference in effectiveness between the two amounts, yet when the AREDS2 recommendation was published, the 80 mg dosage remained.

While genetic testing was still in its infancy when the original AREDS study was designed and implemented, genetic samples were taken from some of the subjects in the study and were ultimately reviewed. One researcher found that not only zinc alone but also the combination of zinc and antioxidant vitamins may be harmful to people with a specific genetic makeup, and can accelerate the progression to late AMD.

Obviously, a good many questions remain regarding the use of zinc. Many professionals question whether the 80-mg dose is still recommended when the 25-mg dose provides the same result. Others have suggested that patients have genetic testing prior to taking the AREDS formula to gauge whether zinc is likely to exert positive or negative effects on the progression of AMD. (See the inset on genetic testing on page 60.) Because the original AREDS study authors stated that this testing is not necessary, this controversy continues. Taking all study results into consideration, we feel that the lower dose is appropriate.

THE RESULTS OF AN AREDS REVIEW STUDY

In 2017, the American Society for Nutrition published a review article from the Moran Eye Center, University of Utah School of Medicine, titled "The Age-Related Eye Disease 2 Study: Micronutrients in the Treatment of Macular Degeneration." In large part a review of the two AREDS studies, the article examines the science behind the nutritional supplements included in this and other interventional trials and the reasons for considering their inclusion to lower the rate of AMD progression.

The review looks at vitamins, including C, E, B$_6$, B$_{12}$, and folic acid (B$_9$). The authors report that low vitamin C levels are associated with an increased risk of AMD, but that high concentrations are not protective and do not significantly affect the progression of AMD.

The review also discusses vitamin E and its role in controlling oxidative stress, which is believed to contribute to macular degeneration. The authors suggest that vitamin E deficiency could lead to the accumulation of drusen, retinal damage, and the loss of photoreceptors (cones and rods), and that supplementation of vitamin E should slow the progression of AMD. However, it is noted that other studies have found that this vitamin does not appear to protect against *early* AMD.

The review also focuses on a 2009 study which indicated that daily supplementation with folic acid (vitamin B$_9$) and vitamins B$_6$ and B$_{12}$ decrease the risk of AMD in women. This particular study was supported by a ten-year follow-up in the Blue Mountains Eye

Genetics and AMD Testing

More than fifteen genes are reported to be associated with an increased risk of developing AMD, and they account for almost 70 percent of the risk. Researchers discovered these AMD-related genes through family studies and, eventually, through large-scale studies of people's *genomes*—their complete sets of DNA. The genes they identified have been found to influence several processes within the body that are associated with the start of AMD, the progression of the disease, and the involvement of the second eye.

Several companies offer genetic testing and analysis that can help you better understand your risk for the development and progression of AMD. One test called Macula Risk PGx (by ArcticDx) combines a patient's current AMD status, genetic predisposition, and non-genetic risk factors to determine the two-, five-, and ten-year risk of developing advanced AMD, either geographic atrophy (late dry AMD) or neovascular (wet) AMD. The complexity of the AMD disease process is reflected in the large number and variety of risk factors that are considered in the Macula Risk PGx test, including clinical information (such as age and BMI) and fifteen genetic markers across twelve AMD-associated genes.

Study, suggesting that deficiencies of folic acid and B$_{12}$ increase AMD risk.

The Moran Eye Center review does a great job of separating the antioxidant functions of beta-carotene, which is a hydrocarbon carotenoid, and lutein and zeaxanthin, which are the carotenoids found in the macula. The authors point out that under certain conditions, beta-carotene can act as a tumor promoter, as mentioned earlier. They also state that consuming too much beta-carotene can actually reduce the amount of lutein and zeaxanthin that reaches the retina.

As for zinc, they verify that the group taking the high amount of zinc included in the first AREDS study and the group taking the comparatively low amount of zinc showed the same results.

This review confirms that no significant correlation has been found between omega-3 EPA and DHA supplementation (omega-3 fatty acids) and the progression of AMD. However it also states that

---

This test is most appropriate for patients who have been diagnosed with dry AMD in at least one eye. Available only through an eye-care provider, it uses a simple cheek swab to take a sample of the patient's DNA. Most insurance providers will cover the test as long as the doctor has detected drusen deposits in the patient's retina.

The company that offers Macula Risk PGx also offers Vita Risk. This test uses the patient's genes to determine which of the available eye supplement formulations offer the greatest benefit and the smallest risk. (As you learned on page 59, the nutrient zinc may cause problems in people with a specific genetic makeup.)

The RetnaGene AMD test (by Nicox) evaluates the chance that a patient with early or intermediate AMD will progress to advanced neovascular (wet) AMD within two, five, and ten years. This test assesses the impact of twelve genetic variants and determines whether the patient is in a low-, moderate-, or high-risk group. Again, most insurance providers will cover the test as long as the doctor reports drusen deposits.

We *strongly* encourage anyone with early drusen or established AMD to have one of these tests performed. The sooner you know about any genetic factors that can influence AMD, the sooner you will be able to modify your diet and lifestyle to reduce the risk of progression.

the Nutritional AMD Treatment-2 Study (NAT-2 Study), in which patients were administered 840 mg DHA and 270 mg EPA for three years, suggests that the incidence of choroidal neovascularization (the creation of blood vessels that characterize wet AMD) is markedly reduced by DHA supplementation.

The conclusion of this review demonstrates that, based on the AREDS2 study results, the AREDS2 formulation with 10 mg lutein and 2 mg zeaxanthin is now the standard of care for reducing the probability of advanced AMD patients with substantial risk factors for progression to severe visual loss. The AREDS2 trial failed to show that fish oil supplements have any benefits, and the beta-carotene in the original AREDS formula is no longer recommended because of potential lung cancer risks, as well as the absorption competition between beta-carotene and lutein and zeaxanthin.

The authors point out that ARED2 was not designed to determine whether individuals without signs or symptoms of AMD should take supplements, but state that clinicians should advise everyone concerned about developing AMD to practice a healthy, vigorous lifestyle by avoiding smoking, getting regular physical activity, and maintaining a diet rich in colorful fruits and vegetables and oily fish. We fully support this recommendation. It is also important to note that according to this review, further micronutrients—nutrients not tested in the AREDS trials—might be beneficial in the prevention or treatment of AMD.

CHOOSING AREDS SUPPLEMENTS

There is no shortage of AREDS-based supplements or "eye vitamins" out there. Many pharmacies have several shelves full of AREDS supplement in different forms—such as soft gels, tablets, and even gummies—as well as multivitamins that also contain the nutrients used in the AREDS studies. Your eye doctor may also sell nutrient formulas for people diagnosed with or at high risk for AMD. A search of the Internet will turn up even more eye-health supplements.

When choosing AREDS supplements, put on your reading glasses so you know exactly what you are buying. First and foremost, make sure that the product you select follows the AREDS2 guidelines—that

The Safe Upper Limits
of Micronutrients

In later chapters of this book, you will learn that beyond the AREDS formulas, there are many other micronutrients that can help protect your eyes. As you work with your doctor to create the diet and supplement regimen that's right for you, it's important to keep in mind that overly high amounts of some micronutrients can be just as harmful to your health as insufficient amounts.

While the amounts we recommend in this book are considered safe, if you take several supplement products, including combination products such as multivitamins, you may put yourself at risk for surpassing what health experts call the upper limits (UL) or upper safe levels (USLs or ULSs) for some micronutrients. For instance, you might take an "eye vitamin" with zinc as well as a multivitamin that contains zinc, and end up taking more zinc than your body can handle. You can also exceed upper limits simply by taking too much of a single nutrient, believing that if a little is good, more is better.

Do excessive amounts of micronutrients really pose a danger to your health? Too high a dose of some substances can cause problems ranging from nausea and constipation to more serious consequences such as anemia and permanent nerve damage. Determining upper limits is not a precise science, and safe upper levels are constantly being revised to take new studies into account. In Table 7.1, which begins on page 101, we have listed all of the micronutrients recommended in this book, in each instance stating the suggested dose. If you want to take a higher amount of any of these nutrients— or if you find that the supplements you are using provide a greater amount—be sure to speak to your healthcare provider to determine the level that it is safe for you to consume.

It is possible to get too much of a good thing. By carefully choosing your supplements, sticking to recommended doses, and consulting healthcare professionals when in doubt, you can insure that your supplement plan provides the vision protection you need without the side effects you don't want.

it includes lutein and zeaxanthin instead of beta-carotene, as well as the other nutrients used in the trial (vitamin C, vitamin E, zinc, and copper). "AREDS2" won't necessarily be printed on the package, so you'll have to read the label's "Supplement Facts" to make sure that you're getting what you want. Many companies claim that they are using the "AREDS Formula," but when you read the label, you may find that the formula has been changed, and that the company has left out some of the nutrients used in the trials. Moreover, most manufacturers do not bother to point out that the AREDS results do not pertain to everyone with macular degeneration, and that some consumers will not benefit from these products. Remember that the AREDS formula has been found effective only for people in the intermediate stage of AMD, not the early stages.

One common modification made in these supplements is the amount of zinc, varying from 25 to 80 mg, the two amounts used in the studies. Recall that the AREDS study chose the higher amount even though the lower dose was found to be equally effective. We suggest that you choose the lower dosage, which supplies the benefits but lowers potential risks.

Some companies now add *meso-zeaxanthin* to their eye supplement formulas. Meso-zeaxanthin is one of the chief carotenoids—the others being lutein and zeaxanthin—that are found in the macula, where they play a role in protecting the health of the retina. Formed by a conversion from lutein, meso-zeaxanthin is not routinely found in the American diet, nor was it tested in the AREDS study. If you find a formulation that you like which contains "meso," we think it is fine to use it. However, we don't think that you should choose a product specifically because it contains meso-zeaxanthin.

Lastly, some formulas include the essential fatty acids EPA and DHA, which were included in the study, but did not reach significance in affecting AMD. As we discuss in the next few chapters, though, EPA and DHA likely do have value in protecting your eyes from AMD! (See page 95.)

No prescription from a doctor is required to buy these supplements, and Medicare Part D does not cover their cost. However, if you have a condition that can benefit from a specific nutrient and your doctor writes you a prescription for it, your health insurance may cover part or all of the cost. (Speak to your insurance company to learn the details of your plan.) It can be expensive to take the AREDS formula day after day. That's why it pays to look for coupons—check company websites and look for paper coupons in the vitamin's packaging—and to take advantage of sales.

CONCLUSION

The AREDS formula has been found to slow the progression of age-related macular degeneration. While this is a very positive result, it is important to remember that the formula was not found to stop or reverse AMD and did not prove effective for people in the early stage of the disease. Our view is that many more nutrients can affect the disease process, and that the handful used in the AREDS trials is important, but is not the be-all and end all of eye-healthy nutrients. The next two chapters examine further supplements that can help you protect your eyes and wage a more successful battle against macular degeneration.

6

$\mathscr{P}$lant-Based Supplements

Western herbalism is a healing art that draws upon the herbal traditions of Europe and the Americas. "Western" in this context refers to the methods of using botanicals rather than to the origins of the plants, which may come from Asia, Africa, South America, or Egypt. Herbs (leaves) and spices (roots, bark, and seeds) have been employed for thousands of years to prevent and treat various ailments. Knowledge of their benefits and specific uses have been gathered by physicians and herbalists and preserved through both written records and oral traditions.

Modern pharmaceuticals had their start when researchers began to understand the effects of plant-based therapies, and the earliest drugs were largely based on chemicals found in plants. For instance, salicylic acid, the key ingredient in the anti-inflammatory medication aspirin, originally came from white willow bark. Digitalis, used to make the heart medication digoxin, had its origins in the foxglove plant. As time went on, pharmaceutical companies replaced the plant materials with synthetic materials. But today, there is a growing interest in the benefits of plants and extracts. Many universities are studying the use of plant and marine compounds to treat or reduce the risk of cancer, osteoporosis, cardiovascular disease, cognitive decline, and other age-related disorders, including age-related macular degeneration.

The effects of botanical medicine may be subtle or dramatic, depending on the remedy used and the problems being addressed. Because relatively low concentrations of chemicals are found in plants, herbal remedies usually have a much slower effect than pharmaceutical drugs and have relatively few side effects. Just be aware that although herbs may exert their healing powers slowly, they contain powerful substances. That's why you should be just as careful when using plant-based supplements as you are when using conventional medications. (For more information on safety, see the inset below.)

Not all of the botanical supplements presented in this chapter have been specifically shown to prevent, slow, or reverse age-related

Using Caution with Plant-Based Supplements

Herbs are generally safe when used in proper therapeutic doses. However, most plant-based supplements have not been thoroughly tested for interactions with other herbs, supplements, drugs, or foods. If you have a medical condition or are taking other drugs or supplements, consult with your primary healthcare provider before starting any new therapy, including the plant-based remedies discussed in this chapter. If your doctor is not familiar with the supplements, speak to your pharmacist. For example, blood thinning drugs like Coumadin (warfarin) and ibuprofen seem to be greatly affected by different herbs, so if you're taking these medications, you'll want to make sure that the plant-based supplements you're considering won't pose a problem.

Once you have decided to try herbal supplementation, it makes sense to start with just one herb or spice for a couple of days, so that if you have any allergic reaction, you'll know what caused it. If you tolerate the first supplement well, you can add a second supplement. If all is still well after a few days on the second supplement, you can add a third, etc. Reactions of any kind to the specific supplements discussed in this chapter are rare.

Be sure to follow the directions provided in this chapter or on the supplement package regarding dosage. Remember that botanical sup-

macular degeneration. However, they have all been shown to have strong antioxidant and/or anti-inflammatory properties, to improve blood circulation, or to have other properties that can improve your eye health. For these reasons, they can be an important means of supporting your eyes even if you have not been diagnosed with AMD or are in a very early stage of the disease.

TYPES OF HERBAL PREPARATIONS

Over the centuries, the forms that herbal remedies have taken largely reflected the traditions handed down from one herbal healer to another. Now that herbal supplements are available commercially

plements contain powerful substances, so don't think that it's okay to double or triple the dose to get faster or better results. Either stick with the recommended dose or work with a healthcare professional who's knowledgeable about herbal remedies. Whenever a range of doses is recommended, it is advisable to start with the lowest dose and then, if that supplement is well tolerated, increase the dose to the top of the range for maximum effectiveness. Do not exceed the maximum recommended dose.

Be aware that the concentration of active ingredients in herbal crops can change from year to year and place to place. As a result, the potency of herbal products can vary widely. Manufacturers, who are well aware of these natural variations, try to standardize their products so that you get the same amount of active ingredient in each and every capsule that you buy. For this reason, capsules are usually the most reliable herbal products.

Finally, keep in mind that just because a substance is "natural" does not automatically mean it is safe. For example arsenic is a natural element, but it is also highly poisonous. In the plant world, some mushrooms are edible and nutritious, while others can be lethal. So if you choose to take a supplement that is *not* discussed in this chapter, be sure to research it and discuss it with your healthcare provider. If you experience a side effect once you begin taking it, immediately stop use and contact your physician.

in most pharmacies and even many supermarkets, it's often possible to find several different forms of a single botanical. Below is a brief introduction to each of the types of products you may come across.

- **Tincture.** A tincture is a concentrated herbal extract that uses alcohol as the solvent. It can be made with fresh or dried leaves, roots, bark, flowers, or berries. To use an herbal tincture, you can drink it straight from the dropper or dilute it in tea. It is important to emphasize that a tincture should never be used in the eye.

- **Extract.** An extract is basically a tincture that uses a liquid other than alcohol—usually water—as a solvent. Use it as you would a tincture. Like a tincture, an extract should never be placed in the eye.

- **Capsules.** A pleasant, easy way to take herbs, especially when the plant tastes bitter, a capsule generally consists of a gelatin casing filled with a powdered herb. Capsules are convenient to take with you when you leave home. It's a good idea to swallow the capsule with eight ounces of pure water or herbal tea to help insure that it dissolves in your stomach.

- **Powders.** Powders are made of plant leaves, seeds, flowers, or roots that have been dried and ground. These can be added to hot water or stirred into oils depending on whether they dissolve in water or in oil. Powders can also be turned into *infusions* by pouring hot water over the powdered herb and then steeping it for several minutes to extract its active ingredients. Use an enamel, stainless steel, porcelain, or glass pot with a tight-fitting lid to prevent evaporation and loss of the essential oils—the main medicinal component of some herbs. Steep the herb for ten to twenty minutes. Then strain and drink the infusion lukewarm or cool. At first, the taste may not be appealing, but you'll grow to enjoy it.

- **Teas.** Made from dried herbs steeped in boiling water, teas offer a relaxing way to enjoy the benefits of herbs. You can use loose herbs or convenient pre-bagged teas. Note that an herbal tea is much like an infusion except that a tea is generally (but not always) steeped for a shorter amount of time and uses a smaller amount of herbs.

■ **Herbal Transdermal Patches.** Just as nicotine patches can help you stop smoking by providing a continuous source of nicotine that passes through your skin into your bloodstream, herbal patches are designed to provide a continuous source of an herb's active ingredients. However, not all herbs can be absorbed via your skin, and exactly which ones are effective and which ones are not is not clear at this point. Research studies that used herbal skin patches to control cancer pain, diabetes, and osteoarthritis have shown promising results. But until more studies have been performed, we advise you to take your plant-based supplements by mouth.

PLANT-BASED SUPPLEMENTS FOR AMD

There are several plant-based supplements that can help prevent or stabilize age-related macular degeneration. As you will see, most of them are brightly colored because of their phytochemicals— chemical compounds produced by plants. For example, annatto is a bright orange-red color, turmeric is yellow, saffron is reddish, and grapeseed is light purple. The chemicals that give them their colors are strong antioxidants that help fight the oxidative stress and inflammation that occur in the retina and are responsible in part for AMD.

■ ANNATTO

Also called achiote and *Bixa orellana,* annatto is a small tree that is native to South America. You may have seen annatto listed as an ingredient in a variety of products, as its seeds are often used to impart an attractive golden color to foods—particularly butter and cheese, but also cakes, baked goods, snack foods, breakfast cereal, and sausage. In South America, it is ground into a powder that is added to foods for its flavor. But annatto has medicinal uses as well. Both the leaves and the brightly colored seeds have been employed by European herbalists for more than one hundred years. Annatto is prized for its antibacterial and anti-inflammatory effects, as well as for its blood sugar-lowering ability.

71

The intense orange-red color of annatto seeds comes from beta-carotene and two other carotenoids—*bixin* and *norbixen*—that give it strong antioxidant properties. Carotenoids are important for eye health and for preventing age-related ailments such as cancer, cataracts, and AMD. Japanese researchers have reported significant improvement using bixin to reduce oxidative stress in retinal cell cultures and prevent retinal degeneration in mice. In a Brazilian study of diabetic rats, bixin reduced levels of blood glucose, LDL ("bad") cholesterol, and triglycerides, and improved oxidative stress markers. If you are diabetic or prediabetic, you will want to monitor your blood sugar carefully when using annatto because it may affect those levels.

Annatto comes powdered in capsules, which can be expensive. If you do choose to use capsules, however, take 50 to 125 mg once or twice daily. A more economical approach is to make your own extract from the seeds, which you can purchase online. Bixen dissolves in fat, so put 1/2 cup of olive oil in a small saucepan. Add 1 1/2 tablespoons of annatto seeds, turn the heat to medium, and stir the mixture continuously until the oil turns a deep reddish orange color. If bubbles appear, decrease the heat. (If the fat looks brown, you have burned it and must start over!) Strain out the seeds and cool the liquid. Pour the liquid into a small glass container with a lid, and refrigerate. Take 1 to 2 teaspoons of the thick oil once or twice each day. Be careful not to spill the oil, because it will stain porous counters and sinks and is not easy to remove. Annatto will also stain your clothes, but can be taken out using laundry stain removers. Be aware that allergic reactions to annatto, such as hives, have been reported in medical literature. Because beta-carotene is a natural component of annatto, this supplement does not increase the risk of cancer.

■ BILBERRY

The bilberry plant is a small, shrubby perennial that grows in the woods and meadows of northern Europe. It is related to blueberry, cranberry, and huckleberry plants. Bilberry (*Vaccinium myrtillus*)—also known as Tuscan bilberry—has numerous health benefits and is completely nontoxic, having no side effects and no contraindications. The plant's fruit and leaves contain several phytochemicals, including flavonoids and anthocyanins, which serve to prevent capillary fragility, thin the blood, lower blood pressure, improve blood supply to the nervous system, and lower blood sugar. Bilberry also acts as a powerful antioxidant within cells and has anti-inflammatory properties.

European scientists studied the effects of bilberry extract in a double-blind study in patients with type 2 diabetes—a risk factor for AMD explained in Chapter 3. The group taking the bilberry had their plasma glucose and insulin each reduced by 18 percent compared with the placebo group.

Bilberry phytochemicals may have potential for treating AMD. In a study using bilberry extract, researchers tested its effects in human retinal cells in a culture. As you know from Chapter 3, high-energy blue light can severely damage retinal cells. So the researchers exposed the cells to blue light and tested whether the bilberry extract protected them. It did so by decreasing oxidative stress and cell death caused by the light. This report suggests that bilberry extract may offer AMD patients some protection against the effects of high-energy blue light.

Bilberry can be purchased as capsules, extract, or tea. The least expensive option is probably the tea. Just place one teaspoon of bilberry leaves in a cup of boiling water, remove it from the heat, and allow it to sit for fifteen minutes. Strain and enjoy. If you prefer to use capsules or extract, take 60 to 280 mg daily.

■ CACAO, COCOA, AND CHOCOLATE

Is chocolate one of the foods you consume for pure pleasure? As you might already know, this treat is more than just delicious—it has many health benefits, as well.

Ground cocoa contains more than a hundred different compounds and is rich in polyphenols, some of which are strong antioxidants. Cocoa (*Theobroma cacao*) has been examined in depth for its potential to fight heart disease. Studies have reported that a low intake of cocoa is associated with a higher risk of cardiovascular death, as well as all causes of death. In one study, scientists gave one group of patients with pre-hypertension dark chocolate for eighteen weeks. The cocoa significantly reduced blood pressure and increased nitric oxide, which also lowers blood pressure.

Other researchers conducted a meta-analysis that examined data from several intervention trials. The researchers reported that those who consumed chocolate had significantly reduced blood pressure by the end of the trials. In yet another study, scientists found that chocolate reduces inflammation, makes platelets less sticky so they are less inclined to clot, increases HDL ("good") cholesterol, and slightly decreases LDL ("bad") cholesterol.

Does chocolate have any effect on macular degeneration? To date, the effects of chocolate on AMD have not been reported. However, dark chocolate consumption does show promise in reducing high blood pressure, heart disease, and even elevated blood sugar while improving insulin resistance. These are all significant risk factors for AMD, so you may infer that decreasing your risk for these disorders can also decrease your risk for AMD. While research continues, enjoy *small* amounts of dark chocolate each day.

Making Your Own Chocolate Squares

Here's an easy, inexpensive recipe for making dark chocolate that's far more healthy than most of the products sold in stores. Start by buying organic cocoa butter, ground cocoa or cacao, and raw walnuts at your local health food store. Spray a small square cake pan with vegetable oil, and arrange a layer of raw walnut pieces on the bottom. Set the pan aside.

Measure out about one cup of the cocoa butter (it comes in clumps, so you'll have to estimate the amount), and place it in the top of a double-boiler that has been set over boiling water. Turn the heat to low, and wait until the butter melts completely. Add about one cup of the cocoa, and stir until well mixed. Add unprocessed honey or xylitol, and stir until dissolved. This chocolate mixture is pretty bitter, so taste it as you add your sweetener until the flavor is acceptable to you. Pour the chocolate over the walnuts, and refrigerate until firm.

When the chocolate is firm, break it into pieces that are one to two inches across. Eat one or two pieces a day. You'll be getting polyphenols from the cocoa and omega-3 fatty acids from the walnuts. Both the chocolate and the walnuts may also help lower your blood sugar.

It's essential to understand that all cocoa-based products are not equally healthy. *Cacao powder* is made by cold-pressing unroasted cocoa beans. It contains all of the nutrients found in the beans, including fats, vitamins, minerals, fiber, carbohydrates, protein, and enzymes. *Cocoa powder* is made from raw cacao that has been roasted at high temperatures. This process reduces the overall nutritional value of the product, but makes the product somewhat sweeter in taste. *Chocolate* refers to the confection made by adding cocoa butter (the fat that's pressed out of cocoa beans), sugar, and other ingredients to cocoa. While these additions make cocoa creamy and sweet, they also diminish its nutrient value. *Milk chocolate* also includes milk, which further decreases cocoa's benefits, probably because the milk proteins bind to the healthy polyphenols, preventing their absorption. White chocolate has no polyphenols and no known health benefits. If your goal is to improve your health, you want to use a product that contains a high amount of cacao or cocoa, and relatively small amounts of sugar and other ingredients.

To enjoy the greatest benefits of cocoa, you can make your own dark chocolate squares by following the recipe in the inset on page 74. If you'd rather buy ready-made chocolate, look for a product that has a high percentage of cacao and little or no sugar, because that bar will have the greatest amounts of flavonoids. For example, ChocZero 85-Percent Ultimate Dark Chocolate is antioxidant rich and sweetened with monk fruit, not sugar. Alternatively, try Lily's Dark Chocolate, which is 55-percent cacao and sweetened with stevia. Remember, you don't want to eat more than one or two square inches each day!

Chocolate causes problems for some people. Individuals who are allergic to chocolate can develop asthma, skin rashes, and other allergic symptoms. Many drug interactions are also possible. For example, chocolate can increase the risk of bleeding when taken with blood-thinning medications such as Coumadin (warfarin), aspirin, and ibuprofen. For more information about interactions between cocoa and drugs, check with your doctor or pharmacist.

Because cocoa contains caffeine, too much cocoa or chocolate can cause jitteriness and anxiety, although for most people, one or two squares of chocolate a day will not create a problem. Caffeine can interact with many drugs, as well. How much caffeine is found in chocolate? Half of a small dark chocolate candy bar (about 20 mg) provides 24 to 28 mg of caffeine. In comparison, there are 95 to 165 mg in one cup of coffee, 25 to 48 mg in black tea, and 24 to 28 mg in a serving of cola. If even a small amount of caffeine is a problem for you, you may want to skip the cocoa.

■ GRAPE SEED EXTRACT

When wineries or juice makers process grapes, they are left with what used to be considered "waste products"—the grape seeds. Today, however, the seeds of red grapes are used to make grape seed extract. This extract is extremely rich in antioxidants, especially anthocyanins, which have been found to offer great health benefits.

The antioxidant power of anthocyanins is twenty times greater than vitamin E and fifty times greater than vitamin C. Grape seed extract has been used to treat high cholesterol, heart disease, high blood pressure, poor circulation, and damaged nerves. There is also some evidence that it is helpful in the battle against AMD. In a French study, scientists gave grape seed extract that contained lutein and zeaxanthin to mice with age-related cone and rod photoreceptor dysfunction. The supplement prevented damage from oxidative stress from occurring.

You can find grape seed extract at your health foods store or online as a liquid, tablets, or capsules. Anywhere from 50 to 100 mg a day is considered safe and provides a rich amount of antioxidants. Before taking this supplement, ask your doctor if it would interact with any of your medications. There are concerns that grape seed extract can increase the blood-thinning effects of drugs like Coumadin (warfarin), Plavix (clopidogrel), and aspirin.

■ RESVERATROL

One of the most popular nutrients over the last few years has been the "red wine" molecule called resveratrol. The chief biologically active component in red wine, this compound is also found in grape juice, berries, and peanuts, but in far smaller amounts.

Resveratrol has potent antioxidant and anti-inflammatory properties. Oxidative stress and inflammation are known to play a key role in age-related eye diseases, including age-related macular degeneration, and accumulating evidence suggests that resveratrol may have a potential role in the prevention and treatment of AMD.

Several eye-related studies have been published on the effects of an over-the-counter product known as Longevinex, a resveratrol supplement that also contains vitamin D_3 and inositol hexaphosphate (from rice bran), which are said to make the red wine compound more easily absorbed by the body. Published reports have indicated that Longevinex inhibits the formation of visually destructive new blood vessels at the back of the eyes. One of the first studies, in 2013, showed that wet AMD patients who took Longevinex had their vision improve, although the supplement did not reverse the progress of the disease. It is believed that the improvement was due to the resveratrol's antioxidant powers. In a 2014 study by the same clinic, three patients with late stage wet AMD had improved vision after taking Longevinex for about thirty months. More recently, a study showed that the ability of the eyes to adapt to the dark, which is a measure of retinal health, was improved by the supplement, indicating a lessening of the effects of AMD. Further studies, which should include larger numbers of patients, randomization, and the use of control substances, are needed to confirm these findings. But at this time, the effects of resveratrol, at least in this form, appear promising for people with AMD.

If you choose to take Longevinex as part of your supplement plan, take one Longevinix daily. If you prefer to take a simple resveratrol supplement, look for a product that obtains this nutrient from several resveratrol-rich plants, and take 200 to 500 mg twice daily, being careful not to exceed 1,200 mg per day.

Resveratrol should not be taken at the same time as other medications. It interferes with medicines in a similar fashion to drinking grapefruit juice prior to taking medicines. Mega-dosing (more than 1,200 mg) can have potential negative side effects, so remember that more is not better!

■ SAFFRON

Native to Southwest Asia, but now grown elsewhere as well, saffron (*Crocus sativus*) has been used for thousands of years to season and impart a bright yellow color to foods. It has also been used in traditional medicine. Cooks and healers both prize the stigmas—the threadlike portions of the flowers. Because it takes about 150 flowers to produce just 1 gram (0.04 ounce) of dry saffron stigmas and the labor needed is intensive, saffron has the distinction of being the world's most expensive spice. Fortunately, the small amount you need to help your eyes will not strain your budget.

Saffron contains more than 150 active compounds. Some of these are carotenoids that act as strong antioxidants and help delay cell death by inactivating free radicals. Human retinal cells in cultures were studied while exposed to damaging light. When saffron extract was added, the cells were protected from the light's harmful effects. Researchers also tested the effects of saffron on mice that had been exposed to harmful light and reported that saffron protected the retinal cells from damage.

Studies have also been performed to test the effects of saffron in patients with AMD. In a 2010 Italian double-blind placebo-controlled study, researchers gave twenty-five patients with early AMD either 20 mg of oral saffron or a placebo for three months. They then periodically performed special tests measuring electrical activity in retinal cells in response to light. After three months, electrical activity was significantly improved in those patients taking the saffron but was not improved in the placebo group. This same effect was demonstrated again at six months.

In another study by the same group of researchers, twenty-nine patients with early AMD in both eyes were given 20 mg of saffron and studied every three months over a fifteen-month period. As seen in the earlier study, electrical activity improved significantly. In a later study with many of the same scientists, thirty-three early AMD patients were given 20 mg saffron. After eleven months, they showed significantly improved electrical activity, which had stabilized after three months. What's fascinating is that after three months, the participants' visual acuity—the ability to read the Snellen eye chart—improved by two lines and remained stable! All patients reported an improvement in the quality of their vision, including better contrast and color perception, reading ability, and vision under low light conditions. They even reported an improvement in the quality of their lives!

High doses of saffron—more than 1,500 mg—may cause side effects, some of them serious, but using smaller amounts appears to be safe. Allergic reactions can occur with saffron, but this does not seem to be common. Medications for high blood pressure—both hypertensive drugs and calcium channel blockers—may interact with saffron and lower blood pressure too much. Check with your doctor or pharmacist to make sure that it's okay to take saffron. If you decide to try it, it would be prudent to keep track of your blood pressure on a daily basis. A very few patients experience dizziness, worsening of asthma symptoms, and cough.

Saffron extract is readily available in health food stores and is not very expensive. Several supplements contain 88 mg, and although this is higher than the dose used in the studies discussed above, it is well under any toxic level. If you wish to cut costs, order saffron "threads" online. To make saffron tea, place six to eight threads in a cup of very hot water and let them steep for fifteen minutes. Drink as you would tea, and repeat three times a day. Three cups a day of this bright yellow tea will give you all the saffron you need to support eye health.

■ TURMERIC (CURCUMIN)

Turmeric, the "golden spice," is obtained from the roots of the *Curcuma longa* plant, which grows in Southeast Asia. It has been used for thousands of years not only in Indian cooking—curries, for example—but also in Indian and Chinese medicine. The roots are boiled, dried, and then ground into a bright orange colored powder. The powder does not dissolve in water but is soluble in fats and oils, so consuming it with olive oil may aid its absorption. A small amount of black pepper may also increase its absorption.

Curcumin, the most active constituent of turmeric, has strong antioxidant, anti-inflammatory, and anti-tumor effects. That is why it is currently being studied for both the prevention and the treatment of different cancers, diabetes, heart disease, and brain disorders. Data from various studies suggest that curcumin is well tolerated and safe for humans.

What about AMD? Curcumin has been tested for its effects on various eye diseases. In rats that had damaged retinas from light—a rat model of AMD—curcumin significantly improved the retinal damage. In other studies with cell cultures, retinal cells were exposed to hydrogen peroxide, a strong pro-oxidant, but curcumin protected the cells from oxidative stress.

If you decide to try curcumin, you can find capsules at your health food store or online. Several products contain both curcumin and black pepper or black pepper extract for better absorption. We recommend 300 to 750 mg of curcumin daily in a supplement that also provides 5 to 10 mg of black pepper or black pepper extract.

CONCLUSION

As you know from Chapter 2, so far, prescription drugs have not been able to help patients with dry AMD. Moreover, the drugs for wet AMD have to be repeatedly injected in the eye, and may become less effective over time. However, the plant-based supplements discussed in this chapter show exciting promise for helping AMD patients by reducing blood pressure, reducing inflammation, controlling blood sugar levels, improving circulation, providing protection for the retina, and performing other important functions.

If you want to benefit from these supplements, first discuss them with your physician to make sure that you can use them safely. As you know, depending on your physical status and the medications you are currently taking, some of these supplements may be inappropriate for you. Then, as discussed earlier in the chapter, you should introduce them one at a time into your daily routine, using each for several days to make sure that it is causing no ill effects before introducing another supplement.

It is completely up to you whether you take one or all of these supplements, as long as none are contraindicated for you. Although more research is needed to study the effectiveness of these nutrients, they have all been shown to have important AMD-fighting properties. If you take all of them and you find that your macular degeneration is not progressing or is even reversing itself, it won't matter to you whether just one, a handful, or all of these supplements are responsible for your improvement. What will matter is that you are protecting your eyes and improving the quality of your life.

7

*N*utrients for Eye Health

In Chapter 5, you learned about the vitamins and minerals that the AREDS trials proved to be effective in slowing the progression of age-related macular degeneration. These are the nutrients that are found most often in the "eye vitamins" available in drugstores and online. In Chapter 6, you learned about the plant-based supplements that have been shown to support eye health. But many nutrients other than those already discussed are known to benefit the eyes. It's important to remember that the same substances that provide the nourishment needed for overall health—that protect your cells against oxidative stress, improve blood vessel health, work to control cholesterol, and perform other important functions—also support eye health, because the well-being of the eyes is dependent on the well-being of the body. Given the high energy requirement and other special needs of the retina and eyes, certain nutrients are more critical for eye health than they are for the health of just about any other organ.

Can you get all the nutrients your eyes need from diet alone? A healthy eating plan that includes a wide range of wholesome foods is vital for proper eye function. But, as mentioned in Chapter 5, it would be nearly impossible to get adequate amounts of even the AREDS vitamins and minerals from diet alone. Keep in mind, too, that even though Americans have access to the largest supply and variety of foods in the world, all too many of us make poor food choices, and consequently, our diets are low in a number of critical substances.

This chapter discusses the vitamins, minerals, essential fatty acids, and other nutrients that you need to protect your eyes and especially your retina. Some of these healthful compounds were already covered in Chapter 5, and some are being explored for the first time. In each case, we explain why that nutrient is important in the war against AMD. The recommended dose for each nutrient along with considerations for use are provided in Table 7.1, which begins on page 101. Armed with this knowledge, you will be able to work confidently with your doctor to make important decisions about both your diet and your supplement plan.

VITAMINS

Vitamins are organic molecules (meaning they contain carbon atoms) that must be consumed in the diet because they cannot be created by the body. These nutrients contribute to good health by regulating *metabolism,* the chemical reactions that occur to maintain the life of the cells and the organism. Included in these reactions are all of the chemical changes that nutrients undergo from the time they are absorbed until they either become a part of the body or are excreted from the body. Thirteen vitamins are generally recognized as being essential, meaning that they are needed for the body to function—vitamins A, C, D, E, and K; vitamin B_1 (thiamine); vitamin B_2 (riboflavin); vitamin B_3 (niacin); vitamin B_5 (pantothenic acid); vitamin B_6 (pyridoxine); vitamin B_{12} (cobalamin); biotin; and folate.

Vitamins are grouped into two categories, water-soluble and fat-soluble. As the name implies, *water-soluble vitamins* dissolve in water. They must be taken into the body daily, because instead of being stored for future use, they are excreted in the urine on a regular basis, sometimes in as little as two hours. Included in this group are the B vitamins and vitamin C. *Fat-soluble vitamins* dissolve in fat rather than water, and are stored in the body's fatty tissue and liver. They include vitamins A, D, E, and K. Your body needs both water-soluble and fat-soluble vitamins to perform normally, and some vitamins are especially important to the normal functioning of the retina. In the pages that follow, we will look at the most important vitamins for eye health. To find recommended doses and considerations for use, turn to Table 7.1, which begins on page 101.

■ VITAMIN A AND THE CAROTENOIDS

Vitamin A, a fat-soluble vitamin, has many functions in the body. For instance, it helps form and preserve healthy skin, teeth, skeletal and soft tissue, and the mucous membranes. Vitamin A is also crucial to the maintenance of eye health. As a powerful antioxidant, it is involved in reducing inflammation and fighting free-radical damage, both of which contribute to AMD. It is also needed to help the retina produce pigments that protect it from light, and it is an integral part of the transformation of light energy into nerve impulses, a process that permits images to reach the brain.

Our diet provides two types of vitamin A. One group, called *retinoids,* comes from animal sources. This type of vitamin A is *preformed*—in other words, it is ready for use by the body. Because vitamin A is fat-soluble and not readily excreted from the body, it can accumulate and create an imbalance, which could become toxic when doses are extremely large.

The second class of vitamin A provided by the diet is known as the *carotenoids.* These nutrients come from plants. There are over sixty carotenoids found in food, the most famous of which is beta-carotene. Of all the carotenoids, only a few of them—beta-carotene included— are converted by the body into active vitamin A, and then act like pre-formed vitamin A. (The other carotenoids also have important functions in the body.) As you learned in Chapter 5, beta-carotene is a controversial subject in the treatment of macular degeneration. This nutrient can act as an antioxidant that may help protect the retina from oxidative stress, but too much beta-carotene taken as supplements has been linked to lung cancer in both smokers and former smokers, which is why the second AREDS trial replaced beta-carotene with other antioxidants. While several studies have reported that beta-carotene does not affect the risk for AMD, other scientists have found that increased consumption and blood levels of beta-carotene do reduce the risk for wet AMD. Other researchers report that elderly Japanese men with late AMD have significantly lower blood levels of beta-carotene than people who do not have this disorder. Unfortunately, many nutritional supplements use beta-carotene as their source of vitamin A. In some cases, this can cause excess beta-carotene to build up and reduce the amount of protective pigment in the retina by displacing lutein and zeaxanthin, which are major components of the macular pigment.

It is usually better to get beta-carotene from nutrient-packed food sources, such as carrots; sweet potatoes; sweet red peppers; winter squash; spinach, kale, and other dark green leafy vegetables; cantaloupe; and dried apricots. However, to make sure that you get enough vitamin A and beta-carotene, we recommend taking a supplement that pairs pre-formed vitamin A with mixed carotenoids, which include moderate amounts of beta-carotene as well as other important nutrients, such as lycopene.

■ THE B VITAMINS

The nutrients known as the B-complex vitamins are grouped together based on their common sources, their close relationship in vegetable and animal tissue, and their functional relationship. These water-soluble substances include vitamins B_1 (thiamine), B_2 (riboflavin), B_3 (niacin), B_5 (pantothenic acid), B_6 (pyridoxine), B_{12} (cobalamin), biotin, choline, folate, inositol, and para-aminobenzoic acid (PABA). The B vitamins are found naturally in meat, dairy, leafy greens, peas, and whole grains.

The key role of the B vitamins is to provide the body with energy by converting carbohydrates into glucose, which the body uses as fuel. These nutrients are also vital in the metabolism of fats and protein, and are necessary for the normal functioning of the nervous system. In fact, they may be the single most important factor in nerve health. They are essential for the maintenance of muscle tone in the gastrointestinal tract and for the health of the skin, hair, mouth, and liver. Moreover, these vitamins are essential for the health of the eyes.

As first discussed in Chapter 5 (see page 60), the B vitamins have been found to play an important role in combating AMD. A study published in the *Archives of Internal Medicine* demonstrated that women who took vitamin B_6, vitamin B_{12}, and folic acid (B_9) for several years had a significantly lower risk (35 to 40 percent) of developing AMD than same-age women who took a placebo. Researchers hypothesized that the nutrients might have lowered the risk of AMD by decreasing the body's level of homocysteine, a chemical that is synthesized in the body. Patients with dry or wet AMD—as well as heart disease, vascular disease, and other inflammatory disorders—often have elevated levels of homocysteine, which damages blood vessels through inflammation. Vitamins B_6, B_{12}, and folic acid play key roles in converting homocysteine to the amino acid methionine, one of the body's building blocks of new proteins. Without the right amounts of these B vitamins, this conversion is inefficient, and homocysteine builds up.

Although the study mentioned above highlights three members of the B complex, it's essential to recognize that all of the B vitamins should be taken together. Nowhere in nature do we find a single B vitamin isolated from the rest, and there's a reason for that. The B vitamins are so interrelated in function that a large dose of just one of them may be therapeutically valueless or cause a deficiency of other B vitamins.

Because of the water-solubility of the B-complex vitamins, any excess is excreted rather than stored. Therefore, these nutrients must be consumed on a daily basis. Unfortunately, modern Western diets often don't provide enough of the B complex, because these diets are high in processed foods rather than vitamin B-rich whole grains and greens. Moreover, a number of different factors that are common in modern life—including dietary sugar, alcohol, and even sleeping pills—can destroy B vitamins in the digestive tract.

By following the Anti-AMD Diet (see Chapter 10), you will get a rich supply of B vitamins. To insure that you get all the B vitamins needed to combat AMD, we recommend that you also take a B-complex supplement as directed in Table 7.1. (See page 101.) Because these nutrients are water-soluble, there is little chance of overdosing on them.

■ VITAMIN C

Vitamin C, or ascorbic acid, is a water-soluble vitamin and antioxidant that performs a number of important functions in the body. This nutrient builds and maintains collagen, a protein necessary for the formation of the connective tissue in the skin, ligaments, bones, sclera (the white outer layer of the eye), and capillaries. It also plays a role in the healing of wounds and burns and the building of red blood cells. And it supports the immune system, helping to protect us from viral and bacterial infections and improving the body's response to allergies. Fortunately, this nutrient is found in high amounts in a number of fruits and vegetables, including oranges, kiwi, papayas, berries, tomatoes, bell peppers, broccoli, dark leafy greens, and green peas.

Because vitamin C is a powerful antioxidant, it has long been regarded as an ally in the war against age-related macular degeneration. As you learned in Chapter 5, vitamin C was included in both

Antioxidants and Free Radicals

Throughout this book, we discuss nutrients that are important to an anti-AMD program because they are antioxidants. But what exactly are antioxidants, and why are they so valuable? To understand this, you have to learn a little about free radicals and oxidative stress.

A *free radical* is a highly reactive, unstable molecule that has one or more unpaired electrons in the outer ring. To stabilize itself, a free radical seeks out and grabs an electron from a stable compound. This, in turn, creates a new free radical. A chain reaction begins as free radicals run around snatching electrons from other molecules in a process known as *oxidation*.

Free radicals are an inevitable part of normal metabolic processes. These unstable molecules can also form when toxic chemicals such as tobacco smoke enter the body. The exchange of electrons that free radicals cause is harmless as long as it is brief and tightly controlled. But when too many free radicals are present, damage is caused to cells and tissues. A common site of free radical attack is the essential fatty acids in cell membranes. (You'll learn about essential fatty acids on page 95.) This can alter the structure and function of the cell so that the mem-

AREDS trials, where—along with other selected nutrients—it slowed the progression of AMD from the intermediate to advanced stages. Although several other studies did not find a relationship between vitamin C intake or blood levels and the occurrence of early or late AMD, a few smaller trials did indicate an association. One small study of Italian patients showed that subjects with late AMD had significantly lower blood levels of vitamin C than subjects with early AMD. Another study of fifty-six patients with AMD found significantly decreased blood vitamin C levels compared with control subjects.

Because vitamin C is water soluble, it's important to eat vitamin C-rich foods several times a day. Studies have confirmed that vitamin C is flushed from the body in less than three hours, so it should be consumed often. If you take a daily AREDS supplement as well, it will help insure that your body is able to reap the benefits of this important nutrient.

brane is no longer able to transport nutrients, oxygen, and water into the cell, or to regulate the removal of waste products. Continued free radical attacks can rupture the cell membrane, causing the loss of the cellular components and rendering the cell useless. The chemicals in the cell leak into and damage the surrounding tissues. This process is associated with numerous disorders, including arthritis, cancer, Alzheimer's disease, cardiovascular disease, and AMD. In AMD, free radicals cause major damage to the retina's tiny blood vessels, leading to leaky membranes, cell destruction, and eventually, vision loss.

We depend on special enzymes manufactured by the body and on natural chemicals in our foods called *antioxidants* to neutralize free radicals so that they are unable to do harm. Vitamins such as C and E; carotenoids such as beta-carotene; minerals such as zinc; herbs such as bilberry; and other nutrients help defend the body—including the delicate retina—from damage. It's important to understand, though, that antioxidants can be easily used up or depleted. That's why it is crucial to eat a nutrient-rich diet that provides an abundance of antioxidants and, when our diet fails to provide adequate amounts of these healthful compounds, to take supplements that support the body's power to avoid free-radical damage.

■ VITAMIN D

You are probably aware of the important role vitamin D plays in building strong bones and teeth by facilitating the absorption and metabolism of calcium and phosphorus. Moreover, low levels of vitamin D have been associated with hypertension, heart disease, cancer, gum disease, and autism. Vitamin D is thought to affect the activation of more than 200 genes! It is indirectly involved in the manufacture of neurotransmitters such as dopamine and serotonin, which help conduct the nerve impulses that communicate information throughout the brain and body. It also helps protect against infections like colds. Perhaps most important to our discussion, vitamin D has anti-inflammatory properties that appear to make it important in the prevention and slowing of AMD.

Scientists have reported that low plasma levels of vitamin D are associated with early AMD, and that higher blood concentrations seem to reduce the risk of AMD. In fact, in women younger than seventy-five years of age who have high blood vitamin D concentrations, there is a *48-percent decrease in the odds of developing early AMD*. This is astounding!

Vitamin D is provided by just a few foods. It is found in vitamin D-fortified milk, yogurt, margarine, and orange juice; and it occurs naturally in egg yolks, liver, and oily fish. The body produces Vitamin D when sunshine strikes the skin, but with the current emphasis on less sun exposure because of skin cancer concerns, many Americans avoid the sun or use sunscreen, which greatly decreases the amount of vitamin D manufactured by the body. Considering these factors, perhaps it should not come as a surprise that even though this nutrient is fat soluble and can be stored in the body, more than 75 percent of US teens and adults are deficient in vitamin D.

Your doctor can easily measure your blood vitamin D level. If your blood levels are low, you can spend fifteen to twenty minutes a day in the sun without covering your arms and face with sunscreen or a hat. (Dark skin needs more time, and fair skin should get less time.) However, you definitely want to *avoid sunburn*, which can cause skin cancer. And don't forget to wear your sunglasses to protect your eyes from the sun's rays! If your vitamin D levels are found to be low, it is likely that your doctor will also recommend that you take supplements of vitamin D_3, which is stronger and more effective than vitamin D_2. Ask your doctor to recheck your vitamin D in two or three months to see if your levels have increased substantially or if your dose needs to be adjusted.

■ VITAMIN E

Vitamin E, a fat-soluble vitamin, is composed of two groups of compounds called tocopherols and tocotrienols. Four forms of each—alpha, beta, gamma, and delta—exist in nature. Of these various forms, alpha tocopherol is the most active form of vitamin E in humans. Vitamin E is a strong antioxidant that protects all cells, tissues, and organs, including your eyes, from oxidative stress. In particular, vitamin E decreases free radicals formed by oxidation of essential fatty acids (EFAs). (You will learn more about EFAs on page 95 of this chapter.) In your eyes, essential fatty acids form the cell membranes of your retina. These membranes are constantly bombarded by light, resulting in free radicals that damage the retinal cells if not neutralized by antioxidants. Vitamin E also helps provide protection against the damaging effects of many environmental poisons in the air, food, and water, including those in tobacco smoke.

Like vitamin C, discussed earlier in the chapter, vitamin E was used in both AREDS trials because of its strong antioxidant properties. Those trials showed that when Vitamin E is taken with several other nutrients, it can slow the progression of AMD from the intermediate to late stages. A growing body of evidence also shows that increased vitamin E can reduce the risk of AMD. In a few small studies, doctors reported that blood levels of vitamin E were significantly lower in patients with late AMD than they were in patients with early AMD and in controls. In two larger studies, individuals with the highest levels of vitamin E had a reduced risk for signs of both early and late AMD.

Foods high in vitamin E include almonds, spinach, sweet potatoes, avocados, wheat germ, butternut squash, and olive oil. Taking an AREDS2 supplement on a daily basis will help insure that your eyes get the vitamin E they need for good health.

MINERALS

A mineral is a naturally occurring substance that is solid and *inorganic*, meaning it does not contain carbon. The body needs certain minerals in order to function, and since it can't produce these substances, minerals must be consumed in food or as supplements.

Minerals are divided into two groups. *Macrominerals* are needed by the body in large amounts. They include calcium, chloride, magnesium, phosphorus, potassium, sodium, and sulfur. *Microminerals*, on the other hand, are needed by the body in small amounts, which is why they are also referred to as *trace minerals*. They include chromium, cobalt, copper, fluoride, iodine, iron, manganese, molybdenum, selenium, and zinc. It should be noted that the amount needed in the body is not an indication of a mineral's importance.

The discussions that follow provide information on the minerals that are most vital for eye health. To find recommended doses and cautions regarding use, turn to Table 7.1, which begins on page 101.

Toxic Minerals

While some minerals are essential for good health—and some are especially important for well-functioning eyes—there are minerals that not only have no known function in the body, but actually pose a threat to our well-being. Two such minerals are lead and cadmium.

Lead is perhaps the best known toxic mineral. Nearly everyone has heard about the dangers of lead paint and lead-contaminated water. In the body, lead sticks to red blood cells and then moves into soft tissues, like the liver. When cells in the brain absorb lead, the mineral can affect the areas responsible for learning and memory, abstract thought, planning, and attention. Although lead is especially dangerous to children, whose brains are still developing, it is also toxic to adults and can cause harm wherever it lands in the body—including the eyes. It has been found that exposure to this mineral may increase the risk of macular degeneration. Studies have shown that the levels of lead in the retinal tissues of patients with AMD are significantly higher than the levels found in healthy patients.

■ CHROMIUM

Chromium is a trace mineral. Needed only in small amounts, it stimulates the activity of enzymes that are essential in carbohydrate, lipid, and protein metabolism. It is involved in the breakdown of glucose, and also appears to enhance the effectiveness of insulin, thereby increasing the transport of glucose into the cells. Because of its role in glucose metabolism, chromium has been studied extensively in patients with type 2 diabetes. In a review of fifteen studies on this topic, researchers reported that all studies showed improvements in managing diabetes using chromium picolinate, both with and without standard treatments. For example, in a Chinese study evaluating 1,000 mcg of chromium picolinate in sixty type 2 diabetic patients, a nearly 30-percent reduction was seen in fasting glucose, blood glucose after eating, fasting insulin, and glycated hemoglobin (HbA1c). Since diabetes is a risk factor for AMD and is also one of the top causes of blindness, it seems crucial to make sure that you have adequate levels of chromium in your body.

Another toxic mineral is cadmium, which can enter the body through ingestion or inhalation. This substance is a byproduct of some industrial activities and can contaminate fertilizers, which, in turn, contaminate our foods. But while cadmium is present in food in only low levels, it is found in high levels in cigarette smoke. In fact, the levels of cadmium in smokers are almost double those in nonsmokers, which may explain why smoking is a risk factor for AMD. Cadmium accumulates over time. It is known to cause kidney damage, and it also harms cell membranes and causes oxidative stress in many portions of the body, including the eyes.

How can you guard against the toxic, eye-damaging effects of lead and cadmium? Clearly it's crucial to avoid lead-polluted water and lead paint. You can keep your cadmium levels down by eating organic foods, which have half as much cadmium as conventionally grown crops, and by avoiding cigarette smoke. It's also important to know that sufficient amounts of calcium, iron, and zinc are essential for reducing levels of these toxic minerals.

Chromium is found in a variety of foods, including vegetables, fruits, meats, and seafood, but most of these sources contain only small amounts of the nutrient. The foods highest in chromium include shellfish, pears, Brazil nuts, and tomatoes. Supplemental chromium is helpful in insuring that you get an adequate supply of this mineral.

■ COPPER

Although required in only trace amounts, this mighty micromineral performs a variety of important functions. It aids in energy production, assists thyroid function, decreases inflammation, enhances heart health, serves as a component of enzymes, and does much more. One of its many roles is to scavenge free radicals that can damage cells and tissues throughout the body, including the eyes. Studies have shown that levels of copper (and zinc) are significantly lower in the retinas of patients with AMD than they are in the retinas of patients without AMD. As you learned in Chapter 5, copper was used in both AREDS formulas. This inclusion was probably due to its antioxidant powers as well as the need to balance the zinc in the formulas. (Copper deficiency can occur if zinc is taken without copper. See page 58.)

The foods highest in copper are liver and oysters, but this mineral is also found in nuts and seeds, legumes, cherries, avocados, eggs, whole grains, and poultry. Because most common foods contain only a small amount of copper, supplementation is usually required to make sure that you get the copper you need. If you take the AREDS formula, you are getting all the copper your body requires. If not, you should consider taking supplements of both copper and zinc. Just be aware that you should never overdo copper supplementation, because when taken in excess, copper is toxic to the eyes, brain, kidneys, and liver.

■ MAGNESIUM

A macromineral, magnesium is needed by the body in relatively large amounts. Nearly 70 percent of the body's supply is found in the bones, together with calcium and phosphorus, while 30 percent is found in soft tissues and body fluids. On the cellular level, most of the body's magnesium is concentrated in the cells' energy-producing mitochondria, where it activates enzymes necessary for the break-down of fats, carbohydrates, and amino acids. Magnesium also helps to promote the absorption and metabolism of other minerals, as well as the utilization of the B vitamins and vitamins C and E. It is nec-essary for the proper functioning of the nerves and muscles, and it helps to regulate the acid-alkaline balance in the body. It has also been shown to lower blood pressure and improve blood flow. More-over, magnesium helps the body maintain proper blood sugar levels. Because hypertension and elevated blood sugar are risk factors for AMD, it makes sense that obtaining sufficient magnesium is import-ant for eye health.

Foods high in magnesium include dark leafy greens, almonds, pumpkin seeds, whole grains, beans, fish, avocados, bananas, and yogurt. Despite this mineral's presence in many food sources, the typ-ical American diet does not provide an adequate amount, probably because the Western diet is low in healthful whole foods. Moreover, because the body requires and uses magnesium for so many func-tions, it's easy to deplete your stores of this nutrient. For this reason, it may be prudent to take magnesium supplements. However, if you have kidney disease—which can prevent your body from eliminat-ing excess amounts of this mineral—be sure to speak to your doctor about your magnesium needs.

■ POTASSIUM

Like magnesium, potassium is a macromineral and one of the most common elements in the body. Not surprisingly, this mineral has many important functions. It preserves cell structure, maintains acid-base balance, transmits electrical signals between cells and nerves, and is used in glucose and glycogen metabolism. It also helps man-age blood pressure by lessening the effects of sodium (which can increase blood pressure) and easing tension in blood vessel walls. This is important, because as first explained on page 33, high blood pressure can lead to bleeding in the eye, the death of nerve cells, and other problems that can result in retinal damage and vision loss.

Unless your doctor prescribes potassium supplements, it is best to get this nutrient from your diet. In general, a diet that provides an abundance of fruits and vegetables will help insure that you get a healthy amount of this mineral. The foods highest in potassium include avocado, acorn squash, spinach, sweet potato, dried apricots, pomegranate, white beans, and bananas. Just keep in mind that you can get too much of a good thing. The potassium-sodium balance is delicate, and too much potassium can cause serious side effects, including a fatal heart rhythm. So eat lots of produce, and if you have kidney disease—which can prevent your body from eliminating excess amounts of this mineral—be sure to speak to your doctor about your potassium needs.

■ ZINC

Although this micromineral is needed in only small amounts, zinc plays a multitude of roles in the body. It is a constituent of at least twenty-five enzymes involved in digestion and metabolism. It is related to the normal absorption and action of vitamins, especially vitamin A and the B vitamins. It is necessary to break down alcohol and digest carbohydrates. It plays a critical role in general growth and development, and it decreases the body's need for insulin. It is an antioxidant and also has anti-inflammatory effects. The list of zinc's functions goes on and on.

As discussed in Chapter 5, zinc was included in the AREDS formulas because it is known to benefit the eyes by transporting vitamin A into the retina. In the two AREDS trials, when zinc was consumed with a "cocktail" of other eye-healthy nutrients, it slowed the progression of AMD from the intermediate to late stages of the disease. Other studies have supported the positive effects of zinc on eye health. For instance, researchers in New Orleans reported that giving a 25 mg zinc supplement to patients with dry AMD led to significantly improved vision and contrast sensitivity after six months, while the placebo group experienced no improvement.

A wide variety of foods contain zinc. Oysters, red meat, and poultry are the richest sources, but other good sources include beans, nuts, whole grains, dairy products, and fortified breakfast cereals. If you are taking an AREDS eye supplement, you are getting all the zinc you need for good eye health. Some experts, in fact, feel that the AREDS formula supplies too much zinc! (See the discussion that begins on page 58.) However, an AREDS formula has the benefit of pairing zinc with copper. This is important, as zinc and copper compete for absorption, and if zinc is taken without copper, the body may experience copper deficiency.

ESSENTIAL FATTY ACIDS

Over the last few years, there has been a great deal of debate about dietary fats. For instance, experts first demonized saturated fats, saying that they cause heart disease, and later said that these fats weren't quite the villains they were previously believed to be. Fortunately, health experts agree on one indisputable point: *The fats known as essential fatty acids (EFAs) are not only good for you but also necessary for optimal health.* Moreover, these fats, when chosen carefully, can help protect you from age-related macular degeneration.

Essential fatty acids are termed "essential" because they are required for good health but cannot be made by the body, and therefore must be consumed in foods or supplements. There are two types of EFAs: omega-3 and omega-6 fatty acids.

Omega-3 fatty acids—the most famous of which are EPA (eicosapentaenoic acid) and DHA (docosahexaenoic acid)—are the building blocks of all cell membranes. They keep the watery material around the cell separate from the watery contents of the cell, and they are also responsible for the structural integrity of each cell's components. That is why fatty acids play critical roles in the cell membranes of the eye, especially the retina and macula. Omega-3s also are anti-inflammatory and antioxidant in their effects. They reduce the risk of blood clots by preventing platelets from sticking together, and they reduce blood pressure by helping the blood vessel walls to relax. The other group of EFAs, *omega-6 fatty acids,* tend to have the opposite effect of omega-3s. For instance, while omega-3s help reduce inflammation, some omega-6s tend to promote inflammation. They also increase blood clotting and blood pressure.

While it may seem that omega-3s are beneficial and omega-6s are harmful, the body actually needs both groups of EFAs to function properly. For instance, the inflammation that can be associated with omega-6s is an important component of the immune response, and when we suffer cuts and lacerations, we need omega-6s to help our blood clot. Humans are thought to have evolved on a diet that provided a 1-to-1 ratio of omega-6s and omega-3s, and the optimal ratio is thought to be 4 to 1 or lower. But modern Western diets typically have ratios as high as 30 to 1. Why? Omega-6 fatty acids are found in almost everything we eat that contains fat, including fatty meat and poultry, most vegetable oils and products made with vegetable oils (mayonnaise, salad dressings, and fast foods), dairy products, and eggs. Soybean oil, which is rich in omega-6s, is found in most of the processed foods that Americans favor. Omega-3s, however, are found in fatty fish, such as mackerel and salmon, and in dark leafy greens, hemp seeds, flaxseeds, walnuts, Brazil nuts, and a few other foods that Americans tend to eat in small amounts or not at all. It's easy to understand why we consume far more omega-6s than omega-3s. This imbalance is believed to be one of the chief causes of our epidemic of inflammation-related diseases, including macular degeneration.

In light of the benefits provided by omega-3 fatty acids and the fact that our diets are woefully low in these EFAs, researchers have tested the results of omega-3 supplementation on subjects with macular degeneration. At least two trials have shown promising results.

In 2015, two scientists from Cyprus reported that patients with dry AMD greatly benefited from taking rather large daily doses of omega-3s—3.4 grams of EPA and 1.6 grams of DHA. Besides testing their vision, the researchers measured blood levels of EPA and DHA at baseline and then at the end of the study. Over five months, the patients' visual acuity actually *improved* by a gain of one line or more on the vision chart! In a later study, the same scientists gave patients with mild to moderate visual impairment 5 to 7 grams of DHA and EPA each day. After six months, the patients were able to read fifteen more letters on the eye chart than they had been able to read previously. Researchers also reported that a sub-group of patients with severe dry AMD and severe visual impairment (they fell into the blindness category) experienced significantly improved vision after just three months on omega-3 supplements. In fact, they were no longer considered blind. Importantly, the supplements caused no side effects. These are exciting results considering that most eye doctors regard AMD as always progressing, never improving.

Supplementation with omega-3s in patients with early AMD and the development of wet AMD has also been studied. According to a 2013 article in the prestigious journal *Ophthalmology*, scientists supplemented participants with 840 mg per day of DHA and 270 mg per day of EPA for three years. This dose was much lower than the doses used in the studies discussed above. The researchers also measured fatty acids in red blood cell membranes prior to and at the end of the study. The incidence of wet AMD was found to be significantly lower in patients who had high levels of EPA and DHA.

The Anti-AMD Diet outlined in Chapter 10 provides a healthy balance of omega-3 and omega-6 fatty acids. To make sure that you enjoy the benefits that these healthy fats have to offer, you should also consider adding fish oil supplements to your daily anti-AMD plan. (See page 103 of Table 7.1.) Just keep in mind that fish oils are natural blood thinners, so moderation and balance are the keys to success.

ANTIOXIDANTS

We have already discussed oxidative stress and the damage it does to our cells and, of course, our eyes. (See the inset on page 86.) We talked about how it plays a major role in causing AMD, and we discussed which vitamins and minerals act as antioxidants—vitamin C, vitamin E, carotenoids such as beta-carotene, and minerals such as zinc. Below we will talk about several other antioxidants that are neither vitamins nor minerals but are involved in protecting our eyes from free radicals.

■ ALPHA-LIPOIC ACID

Alpha-lipoic acid (ALA) is a nutrient that is present in the cells' mitochondria, where it is used for energy production. Well known for its antioxidant powers, ALA can scavenge a variety of free radicals and can bind to metal ions to prevent oxidative stress. This nutrient has also been shown to improve insulin sensitivity in type 2 diabetics.

Studies using the *retinal pigment epithelium (RPE)*—the pigmented layer of the retina—have shown that ALA can protect mitochondria from oxidative stress. For this reason, scientists decided to test ALA's effects on patients with age-related macular degeneration. In one study, researchers gave thirty-two participants with AMD 600 mg of ALA daily for three months, while thirty patients received a placebo. Blood tests performed before and after supplementation showed that superoxide dismutase (SOD), an enzyme that breaks down the free radical superoxide, was significantly increased in the ALA group, indicating that the nutrient was having protective effects.

In another study involving a hundred participants with dry AMD, Chinese researchers gave fifty subjects 200 mg of ALA each day for three months, while the control group received vitamin C. As in the study discussed above, the ALA group experienced a considerable increase in SOD, while the placebo group did not. The researchers also administered a visual quality of life questionnaire at baseline and after three months of supplementation. Only those individuals who had received ALA reported a distinct difference. Although visual acuity was not enhanced, contrast sensitivity—the ability to see in low-light situations—was significantly improved in the ALA group.

The foods highest in ALA include spinach, cow kidney and heart, broccoli, tomatoes, peas, Brussels sprouts, and rice bran. Supplements are also available. Just keep in mind that ALA supplements may cause gastrointestinal side effects in some older patients, especially at doses higher than those used in the studies cited above.

■ COENZYME Q_{10}

Coenzyme Q_{10} (CoQ_{10}) is a fat-soluble nutrient that can be found in almost every cell of the body, where it has the important job of producing cellular energy. Also a powerful antioxidant, it is called a *coenzyme* because it helps the enzymes in the body do their jobs.

CoQ_{10} is important for AMD patients. Because the retina's rate of oxidative metabolism—the use of oxygen to make energy—is high, this structure is very vulnerable to oxidative stress. Moreover, CoQ_{10} levels in the retina can decline by approximately 40 percent with age.

This decline can have two consequences: a decrease in the body's ability to neutralize free radicals and prevent oxidative damage in the retina, and a decrease in the retina's synthesis of ATP, a substance that serves as the energy currency of the cell. Ultimately, the decline of CoQ_{10} production may be associated with age-related macular degeneration.

In a 2005 article appearing in *Ophthalmologica,* researchers in Hungary shared the results of a clinical trial that was designed to learn the effects of treatment with nutrients known to improve mitochondrial function in people with early AMD. Phototrop, the supplement used in the study, included 10 mg of CoQ_{10} plus 100 mg of acetyl-L-carnitine and 530 mg of omega-3 fatty acids. The control group took a placebo of soy oil.

At the end of the study, the researchers found that those who had taken the nutrient supplement experienced improvements along several parameters of eyesight. For example, the participants who took the supplement had a 23-percent *decrease* in the area of their sight affected by AMD, while the placebo group showed a 13-percent *increase* in the area. Those individuals taking the supplement also had an improved ability to read the Snellen eye chart, while the controls had a decreased ability. Finally, special photos of the retina taken before and after the study showed a significant improvement in the retinas of the supplemented participants and a worsening of the retinas of the control group. In other words, this study proved that nutrients can make a big difference to the progression of AMD in people who are in the early stages of the disease. This is of importance to everyone with AMD, and is of particular significance to the millions of Americans who take statins for elevated cholesterol, as statins can reduce CoQ_{10} levels by up to 40 percent.

Foods high in CoQ_{10} include anchovies, beef, herring, mackerel, broccoli, and cauliflower. To insure that you take in a therapeutic amount of this nutrient, supplements are suggested.

■ LUTEIN

Lutein is one of the many carotenoids present in food. Specifically, it is found in dark leafy greens, such as kale and spinach, and in other green and yellow vegetables. Broccoli, corn, and peas all supply this nutrient.

Many people think of lutein as the "eye vitamin" because it is almost always included in supplements intended to protect eye health. Lutein is one of three major carotenoids—the others being zeaxanthin and meso-zeaxanthin—that are present in high concentrations in the central macula of the retina. A pigment that helps give the macula its yellowish color, lutein guards the eye from the damaging effects of light, especially the high-energy light rays called blue light. Evidence points to a correlation between the density of the pigment in the macula and a reduced risk for age-related macular degeneration. (Note that while it is vital to consume lutein and zeaxanthin in the diet or through supplements, at this point, it does not appear to be necessary to take meso-zeaxathin, because lutein is converted to meso-zeaxanthin in the retina.)

Because of lutein's important role in safeguarding eye health and strong antioxidant properties, it was used in the AREDS trials and is included in AREDS supplements. In the trials, when taken with several other nutrients, it was found to slow the progression of AMD from the intermediate to late stages. If you take an AREDS supplement, you may be getting all the lutein you need to support your eyes. Of course, it is also important to eat healthy lutein-rich foods, because they supply other important nutrients that enhance overall health. Moreover, some doctors suggest additional lutein supplementation for individuals who have been diagnosed with AMD. (See page 103 of Table 7.1.)

■ MELATONIN

Melatonin is a hormone that is well known for its role in helping induce sleep, and for years, people have used supplements of this hormone as a natural sleep aid. Studies now show that melatonin might also help your eyes. The photoreceptors in the retina produce melatonin, which is made at high levels at night and lower levels during the day. It is believed that the substance plays several roles in the retina, and as an antioxidant, one of those roles is to help protect the retina from the oxidative stress of essential fatty acids, which are

Table 7.1. Supplements to Prevent and Treat Age-Related Macular Degeneration

VITAMINS		
Supplement	**Dosage**	**Considerations**
Vitamin A and mixed carotenoids	2,000 IU—half vitamin A and half mixed carotenoids— once a day	Vitamin A has the potential to be toxic if taken in large amounts over time. Do not take high doses if you have liver disease, are a smoker, or are exposed to asbestos.
Vitamin B Complex	75 to 100 mg three times a day	Take a B-complex vitamin supplement that roughly contains the following B vitamins thought to be helpful for AMD and eye health: 15 mg B_1 (thiamine), 5 mg B_2 (riboflavin), 25 mg B_3 (niacin), 10 mg B_6 (pyridoxine), 100 mcg B_9 (folic acid), 500 mcg B_{12} (cobalamin). It's fine if other B vitamins are included in the supplement as well, but those just named are the most critical for eye health.
Vitamin C	250 mg three or four times a day	If you take an AREDS2 supplement, you are getting part of the vitamin C you need for good eye health. Use supplements and vitamin C-rich foods to supply the rest. Note that too much vitamin C can cause gas and diarrhea. Also, do not take a high dose of vitamin C if you are prone to kidney stones or gout.
Vitamin D_3	2,000 to 3,000 IU once a day	This is a suggested dosage only. It's important to have your blood levels measured by your healthcare provider, who will determine the proper dosage for you and monitor your progress.
Vitamin E	Up to 400 IU d-alpha tocopherol or mixed tocopherols once a day	If you take an AREDS2 supplement, you are probably getting all the vitamin E you need.

MINERALS		
Supplement	**Dosage**	**Considerations**
Chromium	1,000 mcg once a day	Use the chromium picolinate form of the nutrient, as it has been shown to help control blood sugar levels.
Copper	1 mg once a day	This is used to balance zinc supplementation. If you take an AREDS2 supplement, you are getting all the copper you need.
Magnesium	100 mg three times a day	If you have kidney disease, consult your your healthcare provider for dosage. If you experience diarrhea, lower your dosage. If you experience abdominal pain, discontinue use and see your doctor.
Potassium	See your healthcare provider for dosage directions.	
Zinc	25 mg once a day	If you take an AREDS2 supplement—which contains 80 mg of zinc daily—you are probably getting more zinc than you need. If possible, find a formula with only 25 mg of zinc. Remember that zinc and copper consumption must be balanced. Taking too much zinc without copper can cause a copper deficiency.

ANTIOXIDANTS		
Supplement	**Dosage**	**Considerations**
Alpha-Lipoic Acid	200 to 600 mg once a day	ALA may cause gastrointestinal side effects in some older patients, especially when taken in high doses. If this occurs, try a lower dose.
Coenzyme Q$_{10}$	30 to 100 mg once a day	Statin drugs reduce the amount of CoQ$_{10}$ in the cells, so if you are taking statins, increase the CoQ$_{10}$ dosage up to 200 mg a day.

Lutein	10 to 20 mg once a day	If you take an AREDS2 supplement, you are probably getting 10 mg of lutein. Some doctors recommend 20 mg for people diagnosed with AMD. Ask your eye doctor for a recommendation.
Melatonin	3 mg once a day	Take directly before bedtime in a darkened room.
Quercetin	100 to 250 mg three times a day	If you are taking a blood thinner or antibiotic, consult your doctor before taking quercetin.
Zeaxanthin	2 to 4 mg once a day	If you take an AREDS2 supplement, you are probably getting 2 mg of zeaxanthin. Some doctors recommend 4 mg for people diagnosed with AMD. Ask your eye doctor for a recommendation.

ESSENTIAL FATTY ACIDS		
Supplement	**Dosage**	**Considerations**
EPA/DHA (fish oil)	1,000 mg once a day	Check the back of the bottle to make sure that the supplement contains both EPA and DHA. Typically, a bottle of fish oil supplements states the total oil on the front label and the amounts of EPA and DHA on the back. It is the amounts on the back that should add up to your chosen dosage. Select a supplement that contains some vitamin E to prevent oxidation and spoilage.
		If you are taking blood-thinning medications, speak to your doctor before taking fish oil, which has blood-thinning effects.
		To prevent fishy tasting burps, take fish oil with food. It may also be helpful to buy supplements with enteric coating or to take smaller doses throughout the day.

PLANT-BASED SUPPLEMENTS		
Supplement	**Dosage**	**Considerations**
Annatto	50 to 125 mg once or twice a day	If you are diabetic or prediabetic, monitor your blood sugar levels carefully when using annatto because it may affect those levels. If you would prefer a homemade annatto extract to the capsules, see page 72.
Bilberry	60 to 280 mg once a day	Bilberry fruit and extract are generally consider safe, and there are no known side effects or contraindications. If you would prefer bilberry tea to capsules or extract, see page 73.
Grape Seed Extract	50 to 100 mg once a day	If you are taking blood-thinning medications, speak to your doctor before taking grape seed extract, which has blood-thinning effects.
Resveratrol	200 to 500 mg twice a day	Look for a product that obtains this nutrient from several resveratrol-rich plants. If you prefer to take Longivinex, the product used in several resveratrol studies, take one daily. Do not take resveratrol at the same time as other medications, as it can interfere with their actions. Do not exceed 1,200 mg a day.
Saffron	88 mg once a day	If you are taking medication to lower blood pressure, speak to your doctor before taking saffron, which has blood pressure-lowering effects. Do not exceed 1,500 mg a day. If you would prefer saffron tea, see page 79.
Turmeric (Curcumin)	300 to 750 mg once a day	Look for a product that includes 5 to 10 mg of black pepper or black pepper extract, as this improves absorption. If you are taking blood-thinning medications, speak to your doctor before taking turmeric, which may have blood-thinning effects. If you experience stomach upset, lower your dosage.

critical for vision. (See the discussion of essential fatty acids on page 95.) It should be noted that the production of melatonin declines with age, which may help explain age-related macular degeneration.

To research the effects of melatonin on AMD, scientists first studied human retinal epithelial cells (RPE) in cell cultures. They produced oxidative stress in the cells by exposing them to hydrogen peroxide (bleach) to see whether melatonin given twice a day for three days could reduce its harmful effects. It did, markedly reducing cell damage and death.

Scientists also studied levels of melatonin in both AMD patients and controls without AMD by measuring melatonin metabolites in the urine. Urinary levels of the metabolite were 40 percent lower in AMD patients than in the controls.

Chinese investigators studied the effects of giving 3 mg of melatonin at bedtime to one hundred patients with wet or dry AMD. After six months of treatment, 90 percent of the patients either remained stable or experienced improved visual acuity. Eye examinations showed that the majority of the subjects had reduced macular damage after six months of taking melatonin. In addition, 78 percent reported that both their sleep and their general feeling of well-being had improved. The authors concluded, "The daily use of 3 mg melatonin seems to protect the retina and to delay macular degeneration." Although there needs to be longer studies of melatonin's effects on eye health, it appears to be safe and could be especially helpful if you're experiencing both AMD and sleep problems. Melatonin is produced by the body and cannot be found in foods, but several foods—including pineapples, oranges, bananas, oats, sweet corn, rice, barley, and tomatoes—have been found to boost melatonin levels.

■ QUERCETIN

Quercetin belongs to a group of plant pigments called flavonoids, which give fruits and vegetables their colors. Like many flavonoids, quercetin is an antioxidant and anti-inflammatory substance that slows the aging process. It is found in a number of plants and plant-based foods, including apples, red wine, dark red cherries, berries, tomatoes, broccoli, cabbage, spinach, kale, and citrus fruits.

Because of its strong antioxidant effects, scientists have added quercetin to cell cultures of the pigmented layer of the retina to study the substance's ability to protect cells from hydrogen peroxide. Quercetin had a significant protective effect against severe oxidative stress. In a study in animals, this time using UV light to cause conditions similar to wet macular degeneration, quercetin appeared to protect the animals' retinas from damage. The authors concluded, "It could become a promising candidate for the treatment of AMD." Human studies have not been reported yet, but since the pigmented layer of the retina has been called the first line of defense against macular degeneration, this is a significant discovery.

If you want to enjoy the benefits of quercetin, include an abundance of fruits and vegetables in your diet, especially those listed above. Quercetin can also be taken as a supplement.

■ ZEAXANTHIN

Like its cousin lutein, discussed on page 99, zeaxanthin is a carotenoid found in the macular pigment. As already explained, this pigment is believed to guard the eye from the damaging effects of the high-energy light known as blue light and thus help prevent the cellular destruction that leads to AMD.

Also like lutein, zeaxanthin is found in fruits and vegetables. In fact, the same produce that is high in lutein—dark leafy greens like kale and spinach, for instance—is also high in this nutrient. (See the discussion of lutein for a more complete list.)

Zeaxanthin was used in both AREDS trials, and when taken with other selected nutrients, including lutein, it slowed the progression of AMD from the intermediate to late stages. Although you will find zeaxanthin in any AREDS2 supplement, it is also a good idea to eat produce that is rich in zeaxanthin, because it will provide you with a number of valuable nutrients that you will not find in pills. In addition, some doctors recommend additional zeaxanthin supplementation for people who have already been diagnosed with AMD. (See page 103 of Table 7.1.)

CONCLUSION

This chapter has reviewed some of the more critical nutrients for retinal health, including those first discussed in Chapter 5, "The AREDS Trials," as well as quite a few additional ones. Table 7.1, which starts on page 101, summarizes these nutrients plus the plant-based supplements discussed in Chapter 6, providing recommended doses as well as considerations for use. With all of this information in hand, you and your doctor will be able to create a supplement plan that supports eye health.

But, as you know, there is so much more that you can do to protect yourself from age-related macular degeneration. Part Three will guide you in following the Anti-AMD Diet, which has been shown to not only support good vision but also improve general health.

Part Three

Macular Degeneration and Your Diet

8

$\mathcal{W}$hat *Not* to Put on Your Plate

In a study published in the *American Journal of Ophthalmology*, researchers from Tufts University and Harvard Medical School compared the effects of Asian and Western diets on the development of age-related macular degeneration. The Asian diet was characterized by a higher intake of *vegetables, beans, fruit, whole grains, tomatoes*, and *seafood*. The Western diet was characterized by a higher intake of *red meat, processed meat, sugar, high-fat dairy products, French fries, refined grains*, and *eggs*. The researchers concluded that participants who ate an Asian-type diet were less likely to experience the progression of early AMD to late AMD than those who consumed a Western-style diet. The scientists concluded that "diet plays an important role in the development of AMD."

Unfortunately, AMD is just one of the health issues our Western diet fosters. It also promotes hardening of the arteries, heart disease, heart failure, and stroke. The blood vessels that "harden" are not just in your heart, but, as you have read, are also in your eyes, where they are strongly associated with AMD. Our diet also promotes type 2 diabetes, which can damage the retina and cause loss of eyesight.

In this chapter, we will discuss the dietary components and food additives that you should avoid, along with common foods that contribute to AMD. To help you make smart dietary choices, we will also guide you in becoming a careful label reader who looks at both the

111

Nutrition Facts label and the ingredients list on a product before you consider making a purchase. At first, this task may seem daunting. However, as you begin to follow the Anti-AMD Diet, you will find that it's really simple. Grocery shopping will go more quickly because you will know exactly what you are going to buy, and the price of your groceries will go down because you'll be eliminating the expensive unhealthy foods that now are probably on your shopping list. Most important, you'll find that the foods on your Anti-AMD Diet are delicious and can help you maintain healthy eyes.

WHAT'S WRONG WITH OUR DIET?

Most of us eat what we like, and usually, the foods we prefer are those we have grown used to eating. As children, for good or bad, we ate what our parents gave us. As we got older, we started to discriminate, consuming foods that we thought tasted good, satisfied our hunger, and, in many cases, were convenient to cook or to pick up at a local restaurant or market. Of course, if the majority of these foods had been good for us, perhaps we would have fewer health issues—from heart attacks to diabetes to AMD. But as we know, our poor diet underlies our nation's health crisis.

The truth is that many of the foods we like—sweet cereals and crunchy, salty snacks, for instance—were designed by manufacturers to turn on our taste buds, but offer little to no real nutritional value. In addition, many of these foods are highly addictive, from the fizzy highly sweetened sodas we drink to the luscious desserts we ask for after eating a full meal. And, of course, there is all that clever advertising which convinces us that certain foods will make us happy and socially successful. While that may sound silly, these ads work very effectively to increase the bottom lines of major food companies.

When we are young, our diet usually seems to create no problems, but as time marches on, our bodies begin to suffer the consequences of poor eating. AMD is one of those consequences, and statistics, unfortunately, don't lie. By age fifty, all too many of us begin to experience vision problems due to macular degeneration. And as you have read in earlier chapters, a lack of the right nutrients may be at their root cause. But you don't have to continue to eat the foods that are making you sick. By understanding which foods are good and which foods are bad, you can gain control of what you consume. And by eating a diet designed to avoid the most harmful foods and encourage the consumption of nutrient-rich foods, you can play a major role in maintaining and healing your vision.

THE MOST COMMON DIETARY COMPONENTS THAT DAMAGE YOUR HEALTH

In this chapter's exploration of what *not* to put on your plate, it makes sense to first look at the "bad" food components that make so much of what we eat damaging to our health. A bad ingredient or component is one that "messes up" your metabolism—both the breaking down of food for energy and the manufacturing of substances necessary for life—and makes your organs function erratically or even shut down. You could call these components "anti-nutrients," because they are the opposite of the healthy nutrients we looked at in Part Two. Once you learn about each of these anti-nutrients, you'll be better able to understand which foods should either be avoided or consumed only in small amounts.

■ SATURATED FATS

If you are like most Americans, you eat too many foods high in saturated fats. Saturated fats are found primarily in animal products, including fatty meats such as beef, veal, lamb, pork, and ham; and whole milk and cheese. The fat marbling that you see in beef and pork is composed of saturated fat. Some vegetable products—including processed coconut oil, palm kernel oil, and solid vegetable shortening—are also high in saturated fats. These fats are generally solid at room temperature.

Why are saturated fats considered unhealthy? Decades of science have proven that saturated fats can raise your "bad" (LDL) cholesterol and place you at higher risk for heart disease. This, of course, can compromise circulation and impede blood flow to the eyes, as well as to other organs of the body. Saturated fat molecules also make cell membranes "stiff" because their chemical structure allows them to pack tightly in membranes. When membranes are not fluid, the cells do not work properly. While saturated fats do not pose the only danger to heart health (see page 122), they do pose a considerable risk.

It should be no surprise that high levels of saturated fat have been shown to be a serious risk factor for AMD. As early as 1995, researchers from the University of Wisconsin Medical School published the results of their study of the fat and cholesterol intake of patients with AMD. They found that those patients who had the highest intake of saturated fat and cholesterol compared with those who had the lowest experienced an *80-percent increased risk for early AMD*. That is huge!

How Much Saturated Fat Is Safe to Eat?

The American Heart Association recommends that no more than 5 to 6 percent of your total daily calories come from saturated fat. So if you eat roughly 2,000 calories per day, your saturated fat calories should not exceed 140 calories, or 11 to 13 grams. Table 8.1 gives you some examples of foods containing saturated fats. You can see how the grams of fat could add up in a hurry!

Table 8.1 Saturated Fats in Your Foods

Food or Beverage	Saturated Fat Per Serving	Total Calories Per Serving
Burger King Double Whopper	18.0 g	850
Big Mac	11.0 g	563
Armour Jumbo Beef Hot Dog	6.0 g	180
Small Häagen-Dazs Vanilla Ice Cream	9.0 g	220
Small Dairy Queen Vanilla Shake	14.0 g	520
Large Starbucks Caffe Latte	4.5 g	190
8 ounces 80-percent Ground Beef	17.4 g	574
Large Pork Chop	7.0 g	318

Clearly, it is important to be aware of the amount of saturated fat found in the food you eat. That is why when buying packaged food, you should always check the Nutrition Facts label, which tells you how much saturated fat and total fat are provided by each serving of the product. (See page 134 for information on reading food labels.)

■ TRANS FATS

A small amount of trans fat is made by nature, but most of the trans fats in our food supply come from partially hydrogenated fats, which are manufactured in factories by adding hydrogen atoms to liquid oils and using a metal catalyst such as a nickel alloy to make them solid like saturated fats. Manufacturers produce these fats because they are easy to use, inexpensive, and give food a "fuller" texture and a longer shelf life. Trans fats are used for frying in fast food restaurants and are also found in many processed products, including frozen pizza, doughnuts, cakes, pie crusts, biscuits, cookies, crackers, and stick margarine and other spreads.

Researchers have found that trans fats behave much like saturated fats in the body, but are even more damaging to your health. Like saturated fats, trans fats raise levels of "bad" (LDL) cholesterol. In addition, they lower the levels of "good" (HDL) cholesterol. This increases your risk for coronary heart disease, stroke, and type 2 diabetes. If they plug up the arteries in your heart, you know that they can also narrow the small blood vessels in your eye, leading to AMD.

How Much Trans Fat Is Safe to Eat?

No amount of trans fat is considered a "safe" amount. That's why you should avoid all products containing partially hydrogenated oils and trans fats. In June 2015, based on overwhelming evidence, the FDA declared that trans fats are *not* safe and told manufacturers to remove them from all processed foods within three years. So the trans fats shown in Table 8.2 will have to be replaced with alternative ingredients by June 2018.

Table 8.2 Trans Fats in Your Foods

Food	Trans Fat Per Serving
Burger King Double Whopper	2.5 g
Large Popeyes Cajun Fries	3.5 g
Popeyes Onion Rings (18 rings)	3.5 g
Jays Kettles Potato Chips (13 chips)	2.5 g
Shoprite Theater Style Popcorn, (2 tablespoons unpopped)	4 g
Marie Callender's Chicken Pot Pie	2 g
Blue Bonnet Stick Margarine (1 tablespoon)	1.5 g
Duncan Hines Classic Vanilla Frosting (2 tablespoons)	1.5 g

Always check a product's Nutrition Facts label to determine if any trans fats are present. Be aware, though, that manufacturers must list the amount of trans fats only if it is 0.5 gram or more per serving, so the label can list 0.0 gram trans fats even if a small amount is present. That is why it is also a good idea to check the ingredients list to see if there are any partially hydrogenated oils—a sure sign that the product contains trans fats.

■ SODIUM AND SODIUM CHLORIDE (SALT)

If you have high blood pressure, your doctor has probably discussed the importance of reducing salt (sodium chloride) in your diet. More than a quarter of adult Americans have high blood pressure, or hypertension (that is, a reading equal to or over 140/90), and another 30 percent suffer from prehypertension (120–139/80–89). (See page 44 for more about hypertension.) Not only is hypertension a risk factor for AMD, but excessive salt can harm blood vessels in ways independent of the damage done by hypertension. In addition to reducing your salt intake, it can be beneficial to consume more calcium-, magnesium-, and potassium-rich foods (milk and dairy products), as well as bicarbonate-rich foods (fruits and vegetables), as all of them can help reduce blood pressure.

Adults differ in how sensitive they are to salt intake. In salt-sensitive patients—about 30 to 50 percent of people with hypertension—even small increases in blood sodium levels can significantly increase blood pressure. To determine if you are salt-sensitive, try following a low-sodium diet for two weeks and see if your blood pressure goes down. Begin by reducing (or cutting out) salt when you cook and at the dinner table. Try using Morton's Lite Salt, which has 50-percent less sodium than regular salt, or use additional spices and herbs in lieu of salt. (Note that Morton Lite should not be used by anyone on a sodium- or potassium-restricted diet.) Be aware, though, that about 75 percent of the sodium in the average American diet comes from restaurant food and packaged foods. For example, a single dinner at a Chinese restaurant may come with about 2,400 mg of sodium or more—much more! Just two slices of some commercially available breads provide more than a third of an entire day's salt budget. So if you want to control your sodium intake, you'll have to avoid restaurant meals and check the Nutrition Facts label on every food you consider purchasing.

How Much Salt Is Safe to Eat?

The US Department of Agriculture recommends that healthy adults limit their sodium intake to less than 2,400 mg per day, or the amount found in roughly a teaspoon of salt. In the United States, the average daily intake of sodium is about 3,000 mg per woman and 4,000 mg per man. Of course, an average can be misleading, since some people avoid consuming salt altogether while others may consume double or triple the recommended amount.

Earlier, we explained a number of steps you can take to reduce the salt in your diet. Clearly, it's important to be aware of the foods that are most likely to provide large amounts of sodium. Table 8.3 states the sodium count for a number of common foods.

By looking at Table 8.3, you can see some of the biggest sodium offenders. In some cases—such as tomato sauce—you will be able to find lower-sodium options. Foods labeled "low-sodium" should have 140 mg or less of sodium, and foods labeled "reduced-sodium" should have 25-percent less sodium than the regular product. But

Table 8.3. Sodium in Your Foods

Food	Sodium Per Serving
1 Slice Bacon	137 mg
1 Slice Ham	360 mg
1 ounce Breakfast Sausage	302 mg
1 ounce Potato Chips	175–185 mg
1 ounce Pretzels	359 mg
1 slice Pizza Hut Pepperoni Pizza	400 mg
1 ounce (39 pieces) Planters Dry Roasted Peanuts, Salted	230 mg
1 tablespoon Soy Sauce*	511 mg
1 Veggie Burger	398 mg
1/2 cup Tomato Sauce	642 mg
1 cup Vegetable Juice Cocktail	500 mg
1 slice Whole Wheat Bread	240–400 mg
1 bowl Cereal	170–300 mg
2 tablespoons Reduced-Fat Italian Salad Dressing	260 mg
1/2 cup Cottage Cheese	270 mg

*Sodium in soy sauce varies greatly, depending on the brand, and may reach well over 1,000 mg in one tablespoon.

it's important to read the Nutrition Facts label to determine the exact amount of sodium present. Also be aware that some foods, in addition to loading your diet with sodium, are simply unhealthy. Bacon, for instance, has lots of saturated fats, preservatives, and corn syrup, and generally provides little protein. Luncheon meats, sausage, hot dogs, and ham contain similar anti-nutrients. Potato chips have been fried in vegetable oil that has been used over and over again, creating toxins. How do you avoid these anti-nutrients? In general, the more you stay away from processed foods, the healthier you will be.

■ SUGARS—NOT SO SWEET AFTER ALL

Sugar is everywhere, and as you may be aware, it poses a significant danger to your health. Evidence is growing that this simple ingredient, which appears under many different names, is a chief culprit in the development of many of the disorders that plague modern society and that can contribute to AMD. So that you can better understand this ingredient, we'll first talk about the four basic types of sugar, one or more of which is found in each of the many sugars you're likely to see listed in the products you buy. (To see all of sugar's many guises, turn to the inset on page 120.) We will then discuss why so many of us are addicted to sugar, and how the excessive consumption of sugar impacts our health.

The first of the four major types of sugar is *glucose*, the sugar that circulates in your blood and provides you with energy. Glucose is the sugar that is elevated in the blood of diabetics. Dextrose, by the way, is identical to glucose, but is made from starchy plants, usually corn.

The second basic type of sugar is *fructose*, or "fruit sugar." This sugar is found naturally in fruits and vegetables. The fiber in fruits and vegetables helps slow the body's absorption of fructose so it doesn't lead to spikes in blood sugar. However, when you turn fruit into juice, you take out the fiber and leave in the fructose, which then causes blood sugar spikes. That's why we don't recommend drinking fruit juices. Note that fructose is also found in high-fructose corn syrup. (We'll talk about that disaster a little later!)

Third is *lactose*, or "milk sugar," which is naturally found in milk. Lactose is made of two simple sugars—galactose and glucose—bound together. If you read the Nutrition Facts label on a carton of plain milk, you will see that 13 g of sugar are listed per cup. That's the lactose. Generally, this sugar does not cause health problems unless you are lactose intolerant.

The fourth basic form of sugar is *sucrose*. Commonly referred to as table sugar, sucrose is one part glucose bonded to one part fructose. This sugar is found naturally in some fruits, but we get most of our sucrose from granulated sugar, which is extracted from sugar cane or sugar beets.

Sugar by Any Other Name Is Still Sugar

Below, you'll find the various names for sugar that are found in the ingredients lists of packaged foods. Some products include a number of these names on a single label. Are the manufacturers trying to disguise their ingredients so you don't realize how much sugar has been included? Whatever the motivation, sugar is still sugar. Look for "Sugars" on the Nutrition Facts label to learn what the total content is of a product you are considering for purchase.

- Agave
- Agave nectar
- Anhydrous dextrose
- Beet sugar
- Brown sugar (light and dark)
- Cane juice
- Cane juice solids
- Cane sugar
- Cane syrup
- Carob syrup
- Caster sugar
- Coconut sugar
- Confectioners' sugar
- Corn syrup
- Corn syrup solids
- Crystalline fructose
- Date sugar
- Dehydrated cane juice
- Demerara sugar
- Dextran
- Dextrose

- Evaporated cane juice
- Evaporated cane syrup
- Evaporated sugar cane
- Fructose
- Fructose crystals
- Fruit juice concentrate
- Fruit juice crystals
- Glazing sugar
- Glucose
- Glucose syrup
- Golden sugar
- Golden syrup
- Granulated sugar
- High-fructose corn syrup (HFCS)
- Honey
- Icing sugar
- Invert sugar
- Invert syrup
- King's syrup
- Lactose

- Malt sugar
- Malt syrup
- Maltose
- Maple sugar
- Maple syrup
- Molasses
- Muscovado
- Nectar
- Pancake syrup
- Panocha
- Powdered sugar
- Raw sugar
- Refiners' syrup
- Sorghum
- Sorghum syrup
- Sucanat
- Sucrose
- Sugar
- Superfine sugar
- Table sugar
- Treacle
- Turbinado sugar
- White sugar
- Yellow sugar

Sugar Tastes Great But...

Like all of us, you were born with a preference for things that taste sweet. This started in your mother's womb with the slightly sweet amniotic fluid, which you actually drank after month four of gestation. After birth, breast milk and formula contained sugar, which helped ensure that you "ate up" and thrived. As you got older, you were probably fed many sugar-laden foods and beverages, and your addiction to sugar began.

Food manufacturers ensure that your addiction grows stronger each day by adding sugar and corn syrup to almost everything. Approximately 75 percent of packaged foods in the United States contain added sugar. Regular soft drinks, fruit drinks, energy drinks, and sports drinks are all full of sugar or high-fructose corn syrup. Even the iodized salt that you buy contains a little added sugar. Sugary treats have become part of every celebration, from birthdays to weddings. And for many people, the meal isn't complete until a sugary dessert is eaten.

Can you really become "addicted" to sugar? According to scientific research, you can. Princeton University tested the effects of sugar on the behavior of rats. Rats were deprived of sugar for twelve hours and then allowed free access to a sugar solution and rat chow. They learned to drink copious amounts of the sugar solution. The researchers reported several effects that were similar to drug abuse: binging, withdrawal, depression, and craving. There *is* such a thing as "sugar addiction," and most Americans and other Western societies are "hooked"! This is how it works: When you drink a sugary beverage or eat a sugar-laden food, your bloodstream is flooded with too much glucose; your brain secretes a powerful feel-good chemical called dopamine; and the pancreas releases insulin. Sometimes referred to as a "sugar high," this mixture of chemicals feels great. But as the insulin works to move the glucose into the body's cells, the glucose level falls, and the sugar high disappears. Your body then begins to crave more sugar until you are unable to resist the urge to gobble down a sweet treat. And the cycle continues.

As we consume more and more sugar, it takes a real toll on the body. In the scenario above, glucose is moved into the body's cells to provide energy, but if the amount of glucose exceeds the amount needed to fuel the body, the excess is stored as fat. This is why sugar consumption is a major contributor to obesity. Sugar has also been shown to contribute to the development of cardiovascular disease, fatty liver disease, hypertension, type 2 diabetes, and kidney disease.

One of the ways in which sugar contributes to illness is through the production of substances known as *advanced glycation end products*, or *AGEs*. When sugar molecules in the body latch on to proteins and fats in a process called glycation, the new compound goes through a series of transformations to ultimately form AGEs. When enough AGEs form, they wreak havoc on the body, resulting in chronic inflammation, hardened blood vessels, and a number of other health disorders, all of which are linked to macular degeneration.

As dangerous as the four types of sugar discussed earlier are to your health, *high-fructose corn syrup (HFCS)* appears to be even more harmful. HFCS first became available in 1967, and its consumption took off like a rocket. Consumers loved it because fructose is 1.7

Sugar and Heart Disease

Our understanding of the role of sugar in causing heart disease evolved later than it might have—all because of a study performed decades ago. During the 1960s, an industry group called the Sugar Research Foundation (now the Sugar Association) paid three well-respected Harvard scientists $50,000 to *falsely* report that saturated fats were the sole cause of heart disease. Prior to their report, research had focused on the role of sugars in heart disease.

The Harvard researchers published their finding in the highly prestigious *New England Journal of Medicine*, strongly influencing cardiovascular research for the next *five decades*! This also led food manufacturers to remove fat from their products and replace it with sugars to make products that consumers would buy again and again. This fraud was recently discovered by a researcher at the University of California at San Francisco and reported in *JAMA Internal Medicine*, another prestigious journal. Now we know that as unhealthy as saturated fat may be, sugar poses a substantial danger to heart health.

Table 8.4. Sugar in Your Foods

Food	Amount of Sugar	Sugars Listed in Ingredients List	Calories
1 slice Betty Crocker Extra Moist Yellow Cake, no icing ($1/_{10}$ cake)*	$4^3/_4$ teaspoons	Sugar, corn syrup	160
2 tablespoons Duncan Hines Classic Chocolate Icing*	$4^3/_4$ teaspoons	Sugar, corn syrup, invert sugar, caramelized sugar	140
12 ounces regular Coke†	$9^3/_4$ teaspoons	HFCS	140
12 ounces regular Pepsi†	$10^1/_4$ teaspoons	HFCS, sugar	150
12 ounces Big Red*	$9^1/_2$ teaspoons	HFCS	150
Frosted Cherry Pop-Tarts*	$4^1/_4$ teaspoons	Corn syrup, HFCS, dextrose, sugar	200
$1/_2$ cup Orange Jell-O gelatin*	$4^3/_4$ teaspoons	Sugar	80
2 Hostess Orange Cupcakes*	$10^1/_2$ teaspoons	Sugar, corn syrup, HFCS, glucose, dextrose	200
1 cup Froot Loops*	3 teaspoons	Sugar	160
$1/_2$ cup Del Monte Fruit Cocktail in Heavy Syrup*	$5^1/_4$ teaspoons	HFCS, sugar, corn syrup	100
2 tablespoons Kraft Catalina Dressing*	2 teaspoons	Sugar	90
2 tablespoons Heinz Ketchup	2 teaspoons	HFCS, corn syrup	40
1 cup Ragu Pasta Sauce	3 teaspoons	Sugar	140
1.59 ounces M&M's Milk Chocolate Candies*	$7^1/_2$ teaspoons	Sugar, lactose, corn syrup	240
12 pieces Brachs Jelly Beans*	$7^1/_2$ teaspoons	Sugar, corn syrup, confectioner's glaze	150

* Contains artificial food dyes.   † Contains caramel coloring.

times sweeter than sucrose. Food manufacturers loved it because it was cheaper than sugar and enhanced the taste and shelf life of their products. Soon, HFCS was being used to sweeten not only beverages—sodas, fruit drinks, and soft drinks—but also breads, cereals, breakfast bars, yogurt, and much more. But researchers soon began to suspect that this new sweetener brought with it real problems. Fructose fails to stimulate the production of insulin and leptin, two hormones that normally help regulate food consumption and body weight—and that are triggered by regular sugar. Thus, fructose is believed to play a major role in the obesity epidemic, which has led to increases in hypertension, diabetes, and other major health problems. Moreover, a high intake of fructose can lead to fatty liver disease, which also promotes the development of heart disease and diabetes.

How Much Sugar Is Safe to Eat?

The American Heart Association recommends that women consume no more than 6 teaspoons of sugar each day and men, 9 teaspoons. As you can see in Table 8.4, it is all too easy to exceed this amount.

Our advice to you is this: First, consume no high-fructose corn syrup. Second, consume as little added sugar as possible, with your goal being zero! If there are now a lot of sugar-laden foods in your diet—soda, cookies, etc.—don't try to go cold turkey and eliminate all of the sugar at once, or you may be plagued by anxiety, shakiness, and sugar cravings that go through the roof. Instead, slowly decrease the amount of sugar in recipes, stop buying sugary foods, skip the candy, and don't drink sodas or other drinks containing sugar. Your eyes and the rest of your body will thank you.

■ ARTIFICIAL SWEETENERS

Some people think that if sugar is harmful, it makes sense to choose foods and beverages prepared with artificial sweeteners. After all, the average can of soda packs about 150 calories, nearly all of them from sugar, while the same amount of diet soda delivers zero calories, and therefore shouldn't contribute to weight gain and all its complications. Unfortunately, studies show that artificial sweeteners have their own adverse effects.

First, it may surprise you to learn that consumers who use artificial sweeteners are at an increased risk for excessive weight gain, metabolic syndrome, type 2 diabetes, hypertension, and cardiovascular disease—all of which are associated with age-related macular degeneration. Moreover, a report in the American Heart Association's journal *Stroke* stated that a high consumption of artificially sweetened soft drinks is associated with a higher risk of stroke and dementia. Various explanations have been offered for some of the problems caused by these additives. For instance, non-nutritive (diet) sweeteners may change the way that people taste food by overstimulating the sugar receptors. This may lead people to crave sweetness and eat only intensely sweet high-calorie foods, while avoiding healthy "unsweet" foods like vegetables. Even fruit may not be sweet enough for people used to artificially sweetened fare. Also, some people think that because they're saving calories by drinking diet beverages, they are free to eat high-calorie foods like cake.

Several studies have also shown that saccharin, sucralose, and aspartame cause problems by altering gut bacteria. In one study, mice given artificial sweeteners developed lower glucose tolerance through the alteration of intestinal bacteria. This resulted in an increase of bacterial communities that are associated with obesity, diabetes, and metabolic disease. In another study, healthy volunteers consumed saccharin for one week. They quickly developed altered intestinal bacteria and poorer glucose tolerance.

The bottom line is that artificial sweeteners like aspartame (Equal, NutraSweet, and Natra Taste Blue), saccharin (Sweet 'N Low), and sucralose (Splenda) should be avoided. In Chapter 10, we will discuss four alternative sweeteners that appear to be safe: stevia, monk fruit, xylitol, and unprocessed honey. (See page 177.) But even then, sweeteners should be used sparingly.

■ ARTIFICIAL FOOD COLORS, FLAVORINGS, AND PRESERVATIVES

While there have been no direct studies linking the consumption of food additives to macular degeneration, common sense offers us a potential connection. The fact is these additives have been shown to cause oxidative stress in rats and behavioral changes in children with ADHD, suggesting that they can affect nerve cells in the brain. And, as we have discussed, your eyes are really an extension of your brain. The US Food and Drug Administration has approved seven food dyes for use in our foods, drugs, and cosmetics—red #3, red #40, yellow #5, yellow #6, blue #1, blue #2, and green #3. Food dyes must be listed as ingredients on food products. Despite the FDA's approval, many artificial food colors are made from petroleum by-products, which is not what you would expect to find in your food. Moreover, these dyes are almost never found in foods that are nutritious. Table 8.4 places an asterisk (*) after those foods that have been artificially colored so that you'll be more aware of which processed foods are likely to contain these ingredients. Foods that contain caramel coloring are marked with a dagger (†). This is not one of the FDA numbered food dyes. However, it should be avoided because it increases the formation of AGEs (first discussed on page 122), which are suspected of being associated with AMD. Furthermore, the manufacturing process used to make some caramel colors produces a potential carcinogen, 4-methylimidazole (4-MEI).

Here is an example of how food manufacturers try to fool us. There are at least two kinds of strawberry milk on the market—one is colored with red #3; the other, with red #40. These colors reinforce the "strawberry-ness" of the milk, which also contains artificial strawberry flavor. If you read the ingredient lists, you will see the dyes listed. What you won't see in strawberry flavored milk are "strawberries," because there are none! So read all your labels and avoid artificial colors as much as possible.

Avoid artificial flavors, as well. There are hundreds of these products, and they have not been tested significantly for safety. Also avoid products that contain preservatives—BHA, BHT (which may cause cancer), sodium benzoate, calcium propionate, and sodium nitrite, for instance. Unbelievably, some additives continue to be approved of by the FDA and used in our foods despite the fact that they have been banned in other countries. (See Table 8.5.) Instead of purchasing these artificially enhanced foods, choose whole fresh or frozen foods that contain no preservatives or only natural preservatives such as vitamins C and E.

Table 8.5. Additives Banned Outside the United States

Additive Allowed in the U.S.	Purpose of the Additive	Countries in Which Additive Is Banned	Possible Side Effects and Other Problems
Arsenic	Used in poultry feed to promote weight gain and prevent parasitic infection.	The European Union.	May promote cancer.
Azodicarbonamide	Bleaches flour and conditions dough.	Australia, the UK, and many European countries.	Asthma.
Brominated Vegetable Oil (BVO)	Acts as emulsifier in sports drinks and citrus-flavored beverages.	100 countries.	May cause thyroid issues, birth defects, and growth problems.
Diphenylamine (DPA)	Slows discoloration of apple skins during storage.	The European Union.	Can break down into nitrosamines, which are carcinogenic.
Olestra (Olean)	Used to make light potato chips.	The UK and Canada.	Oily anal leakage and depletion of fat-soluble vitamins and carotenoids.
Potassium Bromate, Brominated Flour	Helps strengthen dough and allows higher rising.	Europe, Canada, and China. The FDA encourages bakers not to use these substances, but does not prohibit use.	Kidney disorders, nervous system disorders, and gastrointestinal problems.
rBGH, rBST	As synthetic hormones, they boost milk production in cows, leading to increased IGF-1 (insulin growth factor).	Australia, New Zealand, Canada, Japan, and the European Union.	Breast, colon, and prostate cancers.

■ ALCOHOL

Because so many people enjoy at least an occasional drink—and some enjoy far more—it's important to know how alcohol consumption affects age-related macular degeneration. Moderate amounts of alcohol appear to be protective against cardiovascular disease, while heavy amounts increase the risk. Since AMD shares a number of risk factors with cardiovascular disease, it seems likely that moderate consumption might help protect the body from AMD. However, alcohol is also a known neurotoxin that can cause oxidative stress in neurons in the brain. As you might expect, researchers have discovered that both the quantity and the type of alcohol consumed are important.

How Much Alcohol Is Safe to Drink?

According to one group of researchers, more than three standard drinks a day (with 14 g of alcohol per standard drink) *increase* the odds of getting AMD. In a review of other studies, scientists also reported that heavy alcohol intake is associated with early AMD.

Other researchers, however, have reported that moderate wine consumption seems to be associated with *decreased* odds of developing AMD. They did not investigate whether the wine was red or white. Red wine is loaded with phytochemicals—including flavonoids, resveratrol, quercetin, anthocyanins, and more—which might explain its protective effects.

Table 8.6. Standard Servings of Different Types of Alcohol

Alcoholic Beverage	Size of Standard Drink	Alcohol Content in Grams and Percentage
Beer	12 fluid ounces	14 g, or 5%
Wine	5 fluid ounces	14 g, or 12%
Distilled spirits (80 proof)	1.5 fluid ounces	14 g, or 40%

If you are going to drink, the Mayo Clinic recommends that women of all ages consume only one drink per day. Men over age sixty-five should have only one drink per day, while men sixty-five and under can consume two drinks. Each of these beverages should be of standard size, as clarified in Table 8.6.

THE MOST COMMON FOODS
THAT DAMAGE YOUR HEALTH

Now that we have explored the least healthy components of our foods, let us look at the foods and beverages that are most detrimental to both overall health and eye health. As you may have guessed, these are the foods and beverages that contain one or more harmful components. And as you will see, these foods may be the very foods you consume every day.

■ SWEET BEVERAGES

Most commercial beverages are a minefield of harmful ingredients. Soft drinks, fruit drinks, fruit punches, energy drinks, and sports beverages are almost all loaded with sugar, corn syrup, or artificial sweeteners, as well as artificial food dyes and flavorings. Considering that both sugar and artificial sweeteners increase our appetite for more sweet foods, it's no wonder that many Americans have an obesity problem. And, as you know, obesity is a risk factor for AMD. Colas and a number of other beverages contain caffeine, which can cause a short but dramatic rise in blood pressure—another risk factor. Colas also contain phosphoric acid, which binds calcium, magnesium, and zinc in your intestine, making them less easily absorbed and used by the body. And the caramel coloring (discussed on page 126) plus all the sugar can lead to the formation of substances called AGEs, which may play a role in the development of macular degeneration.

How Many Sweet Beverages Are Safe to Drink?

Ideally, you should avoid all sweetened beverages, especially those containing large amounts of sugar or high-fructose corn syrup as well as artificial flavorings and dyes. Your best choices are tea and coffee—preferably without sugar and heavy cream—or a refreshing glass of ice water with a squeeze of lemon or lime. If you do feel the need to add a little sweetener to your beverages, keep it light, and replace refined sugar with the healthier options discussed in Chapter 10. For instance, stevia, monk fruit, and unprocessed honey are all more wholesome choices than refined sugar. Over time, try to get used to beverages that have little or no sweeteners of any kind. Believe it or not, you can re-educate your palate to appreciate drinks that are unsweetened. Just think of the money you will save!

■ RED MEAT

Yes, red meat—beef, pork, and lamb—contains significant amounts of protein, iron, zinc, and B vitamins, especially vitamin B_{12}. However, Americans consume too much red meat, which is high in saturated fat and cholesterol, increasing the risk for heart disease. A high intake of red meat has also been linked to cancer, kidney failure, and type 2 diabetes. But what about AMD?

To pinpoint the dietary risk factors for macular degeneration, scientists from Germany and the Netherlands analyzed dietary records from 1,147 patients with late-stage AMD and 1,773 healthy participants with no AMD. They found that daily fruit consumption was protective, but that high red meat intake—and obesity—was associated with an increased risk for late AMD. The researchers could not answer the question of why red meat is harmful. For instance, they did not know if the chief problem was the high amount of saturated fat, the chemicals contained in the meat, the chemicals produced by high temperatures during cooking, or another factor.

Australian researchers studied the association between AMD and the intake of chicken and red meat in more than 6,700 people age fifty-eight to sixty-nine. They used food frequency questionnaires to collect their data in addition to photos of the macula taken at baseline and roughly ten years later. A high consumption of red meat—including both fresh and processed meat—was found to be associated with early AMD. However, the consumption of chicken more than three and a half times per week was inversely associated with late AMD: The more chicken eaten, the less late AMD, and vice versa. In another large study, also from Australia, researchers discovered that grains, fish, steamed or boiled chicken, vegetables, and nuts were associated with a lower prevalence of advanced AMD, while red meat was associated with a higher prevalence of this eye disorder.

How Much Red Meat Is Safe to Eat?

The American Institute for Cancer Research advises consumers to entirely avoid processed meats that are high in fat, salt, and preservatives—in other words, luncheon meats, ham, hot dogs, and sausage. They further recommend eating no more than eighteen ounces of fresh red meat a week (six 3-ounce servings). (We recommend less. See page 172.) Always choose the leanest cuts with very little visible fat or marbling. Ground beef should be 93-percent lean. Pork and beef that have "loin" or "round" in their names are usually the leanest. Beef labeled "Prime" usually has more fat.

Table 8.7. Fat in Three Ounces of Red Meat

Meat	Total Fat	Saturated Fat
Ground Beef (70% lean)	24 g	9 g
Ground Beef (93% lean)	6 g	2 g
Round Steak	3 g	2 g
Sirloin Steak	12 g	3 g
Baked Boneless Ham	14 g	5 g
Pork Chop, small	7 g	3 g
Lamb Chop, small	18 g	8 g

If you are a big meat eater, reduce the number of times you eat red meat in a week, replacing it with chicken or fish, which should be cooked without frying. Also consider adding plant-based protein, such as tofu, to your diet in lieu of meat. It's a low- or no-fat option that's packed with nutrients, and it's delicious when prepared properly. If you go out to eat and want to splurge on a steak, order the smallest, leanest cut available, or cut a larger portion in half and share it with your spouse or friend. In other words, use meat as a side dish rather than the main event of the meal. The momentary pleasure of having a huge, fatty steak is not worth the loss of your vision!

■ PROCESSED AND REFINED FOODS

Any food that has been purposely changed in some way before consumption is considered *processed*. If you think that this word can be applied to a wide range of foods—some healthy and some harmful—you're right. Minimally processed foods include foods like bagged salads, while frozen fruits and vegetables, canned tomatoes, and canned tuna are slightly more processed. Further processed foods include jarred pasta sauces, salad dressings, and other foods that contain additives to "enhance" both flavor and texture and preserve freshness. More heavily processed foods include crackers and deli meats, and premade meals like frozen pizza are considered the most heavily processed fare.

Most food that is minimally processed is not harmful; in fact, much of it makes it easier for us to benefit from foods like salads, fruits, and vegetables. But as foods get more processed—farther from their natural state—healthy nutrients are stripped out, and unwholesome ingredients like salt, sugar, corn syrup, artificial colors, artificial flavors, and preservatives are added. Most refined foods are created for longer shelf life; to look, smell, and taste good; and to be easy to prepare—or to require no preparation at all. In some cases, refined foods may be entirely composed of refined products with little to no nutritional benefits. These are the foods that are truly damaging to your health. They provide no nutrients to nourish and protect your body, and are packed with harmful ingredients like salt, sugar, and food coloring.

An example of a very common processed food is a refined grain, such as white flour and white flour products, refined cereals, white rice, and white pasta. The government requires that these foods, which have been stripped of their nutrition in the refining process, be enriched with niacin (vitamin B_3), iron, thiamine (vitamin B_1), riboflavin (vitamin B_2), and folic acid (vitamin B_{12}). However, these five essential nutrients are just a few of the nutrients that were destroyed during processing. For example, when wheat kernels are processed into white flour, the fiber and nutrient-rich germ are lost, leaving just starch. When eaten, the starch converts to glucose and quickly raises blood sugar levels because there is no fiber to slow down the absorption!

The enrichment process is like being robbed by a burglar who takes your $100, then feels a little guilty and gives you back $10. You're still out $90! You will know if a product has been processed by reading the ingredients list printed on the package. It may say "white flour" or "enriched white flour" on the package. It may even say "unbleached white flour" if they were so good as to not bleach it. Bleached or unbleached, it's still white flour. Thiamine, riboflavin, and other enriching nutrients will be included toward the end of the list. Stay away from all foods and beverages that have unfamiliar chemicals in the ingredients list. If you cannot pronounce it, don't buy it! If the ingredients list is long, forget the food. Look for whole foods instead.

Most breakfast cereals are also processed foods. Some of the brands marketed to children—and often eaten by adults—are made from refined corn, oats, or wheat; high amounts of sugar and salt; and artificial food dyes and flavorings. Like white flour, some are "fortified," meaning that vitamins and minerals have been added, but they are still without nutritional merit.

How Much Processed Food Is Safe to Eat?

Although fresh unprocessed food is always best, minimally processed foods such as prewashed greens and frozen fruits and veggies are safe to eat and don't have to be limited. More processed foods like canned tomatoes should be used only in moderation and chosen with care to avoid added salt, sugar, and artificial additives. Whenever possible, purchase organic brands, which normally contain better ingredients. Try to entirely avoid highly refined and processed foods, including refined grains and the products that are made from them, such as white bread, white pasta, and breakfast cereal. These "foods" are not only void of nutrients but also often packed with ingredients that can impair your health and lead to disorders that are associated with AMD.

READING FOOD LABELS

Throughout this chapter, we have advised you to read food labels so that you can make informed decisions about the food that goes in your shopping cart and, ultimately, on your table. Most packaged foods must offer Nutrition Facts labels and ingredients lists. (Some foods, such as those manufactured by small businesses and delicatessen-type stores, do not have to bear these labels.) By understanding how to read the information provided on food packages, you can choose foods that meet your dietary goals and help support both your overall health and your eye health.

How to Read a Nutrition Facts Label

The Nutrition Facts label on page 135 (Figure 8.1) is an actual label from a popular snack cake. As you can see, the label first states the *Serving Size*—in this case, one cake. Always compare the manufacturer's serving size with what you are actually eating. Most Nutrition Facts labels underestimate what most people eat, and if you consume more than one cake, you'll be getting larger helpings of both the nutrients and the "anti-nutrients" contained in this food.

Below the Serving Size is the number of *Calories* (150) found in one serving. The section below that focuses on fats, including *Total Fat* (4.5 g), *Saturated Fat* (2.5 g), and *Trans Fat* (0.0 g) found in each cake. The information stated under *% Daily Value* tells you that this product provides 7 percent of your total daily fat intake based on a 2,000-calorie diet, which you may or may not consume. When a packaged food contains polyunsaturated and monounsaturated fats—which are healthier than saturated fats—it states these amounts, as well. But this snack cake includes no "good" fats, a sign that it's a "bad" food.

Below the section on fats, you'll find *Cholesterol* (20 mg), *Sodium* (220 mg), and *Total Carbohydrates* (27 g), and under *Total Carbohydrates*, you'll see *Sugars* (18 g). There are 4 g of sugar in one teaspoon, so this product contains 4.5 teaspoons of sugar. When you read food labels, it

Nutrition Facts

Serving Size 1 cake (42.5g)

Amount Per Serving

Calories 150	Calories from Fat 41
	% Daily Value*
Total Fat 4.5g	**7%**
Saturated Fat 2.5g	**13%**
Trans Fat 0.0g	**13%**
Cholesterol 20mg	**7%**
Sodium 220mg	**9%**
Total Carbohydrates 27.0g	**9%**
Sugars 18.0g	
Protein 1.0g	

Vitamin A 0%	Vitamin C 0%
Calcium 0%	Iron 2%

*Based on a 2000 calorie diet

Figure 8.1. A Nutrition Facts Label.

may be helpful to divide the grams of sugar by 4 so that you can visualize the amount more clearly. Note that on some products, like milk and fruit, the amount of sugar may be misleading because these products contain natural sugar—lactose or fructose. That's why it's so important to read the list of ingredients, as it will help you understand the source of the sugar. Soon, the government will require that Added Sugars also be listed. This will make it possible to see how much sugar is a natural part of the food and how much was added during processing.

On many products, such as whole grain bread and brown rice, the grams of fiber may be listed under *Total Carbohydrates*. But like many unhealthy foods, this snack cake contains no fiber at all.

This Nutrition Facts label ends by listing *Protein* (only 1 gram), no vitamins, and almost no minerals. It should be no surprise that this "food" provides no micronutrients except a trace amount of iron.

How to Read the Ingredients List

Now that we've explored the Nutrition Facts label, let's look at Figure 8.2, the ingredients list. Just the length of the list should be a warning that this is an unhealthy food! Simple good foods usually contain only a few minimally processed ingredients, while junk foods tend to be "manufactured" from a long list of components, including several that you would never find in an actual kitchen.

The flour used to make this product is bleached and refined, with four vitamins and iron "ferrous sulfate" added to partly make up for all the good nutrients that were discarded during processing. Four different types of sugar are listed—sugar, corn syrup, high fructose corn syrup, and dextrose. But as you recall from the discussion on page 119, they are all sugar. Next the label lists partially hydrogenated vegetable shortening, which means that the cake contains harmful trans fats even though the Nutrition Facts label lists none. (Remember, the manufacturer doesn't have to list this ingredient unless there's at least 0.5 gram per serving.) The rest of the ingredients are a mystery unless

INGREDIENTS: ENRICHED BLEACHED WHEAT FLOUR [FLOUR, FERROUS SULFATE, "B" VITAMINS (NIACIN, THIAMINE MONONITRATE (B1), RIBOFLAVIN (B2), FOLIC ACID)], SUGAR, CORN SYRUP, WATER, HIGH FRUCTOSE CORN SYRUP, PARTIALLY HYDROGENATED VEGETABLE SHORTENING (CONTAINS ONE OR MORE OF: SOYBEAN, CANOLA, OR PALM OIL), DEXTROSE, WHOLE EGGS, CONTAINS 2% OR LESS OF: MODIFIED CORNSTARCH, CELLULOSE GUM, WHEY, LEAVENINGS (SODIUM ACID PYROPHOSPHATE, BAKING SODA, MONOCALCIUM PHOSPHATE), SALT, CORNSTARCH, CORN FLOUR, CORN DEXTRINS, MONO AND DIGLYCERIDES, POLYSORBATE 60, SOY LECITHIN, NATURAL AND ARTIFICIAL FLAVORS, SOY PROTEIN ISOLATE, SODIUMTEAROYL LACTYLATE, SODIUM AND CALCIUM CASEINATE, CALCIUM SULFATE, SORBIC ACID (TO RETAIN FRESHNESS), COLOR ADDED (YELLOW 5, RED 40). MAY CONTAIN PEANUTS OR TRACES OF PEANUTS.

Figure 8.2. An Ingredients List.

you are a food scientist—polysorbate 60, sodium stearoyl lactylate, and calcium caseinate, for instance. The list ends with two artificial food dyes made from petroleum by-products—Yellow 5 and Red 40. Be aware that the ingredients listed first are present in the highest amounts. On this label, flour and sugar are the first ingredients stated, meaning that the food is made of largely refined flour and refined sugar, two nutritionally bankrupt foods.

You have learned how to read a product's Nutrition Facts label and ingredients list. Although it may seem a little complicated and time-consuming at first, as you examine more and more products, you will quickly hone your ability to tell the good foods from the bad and make the right choices for your eyes. Knowledge is power!

CONCLUSION

Now you know what *not* to put on your plate. Foods containing too much saturated fat; any amount of trans fats; too much sodium, added sugar, and high-fructose corn syrup; or artificial sweeteners, food dyes, flavors, and preservatives can cause a variety of health disorders, including age-related macular degeneration. Avoid these "anti-nutrients" by avoiding highly processed foods. Also sharply reduce your intake of red meat and processed meats, and limit your consumption of alcohol.

You may be feeling a little overwhelmed by the task of overhauling your diet. Changing the way you eat is not easy. But remember that you don't have to make all the changes today. Transform your menus and meals gradually. Use your new label-reading skills to examine the products found in your pantry and refrigerator. Then use up or, better yet, simply discard those foods that don't meet your new standards. If your kitchen starts to seem a little empty, don't worry. The next two chapters will guide you to healthy foods that *do* belong on your plate because of their ability to improve your overall health and prevent, halt, or even reverse age-related macular degeneration.

9

*W*hat Makes a Food Healthy?

In the last chapter, we looked at all the unhealthy components of today's foods and beverages that can lead to age-related macular degeneration as well as a host of other health problems. Then we talked about the "bad foods" that contain these unhealthy components and how to avoid them. You may have been disappointed to learn that you have to give up some of your favorite "comfort" foods and beverages, or that you'll be able to indulge in them only occasionally. But you'll probably agree that AMD is a high price to pay for the few minutes of pleasure you experience drinking a sweetened beverage or eating a large fatty steak.

Fortunately, there are a lot of delicious foods that not only please the palate but also nourish and protect the eyes. This chapter begins our exploration of healthier foods by looking at the components of food—fiber, for instance—that play a crucial role in maintaining vision, slowing down AMD, and even reversing the damage done by the disease. As you'll find, healthy foods not only support your eyes but also provide good nutrition for *all* of your cells, tissues, and organs, reducing your risks for hypertension, heart disease, type 2 diabetes, and cancer!

Now let's take a close look at each of the components—fiber, protein, essential fatty acids, vitamins and minerals, and phytochemicals—that give our eyes with the nutrition they need.

■ FIBER

One very important component of your diet is fiber. Fiber is what your grandmother used to call "roughage." For a long time, doctors have known that fiber can help relieve constipation, but now the medical community recognizes that fiber can also decrease the risk for a number of more serious disorders, including heart disease, stroke, obesity, type 2 diabetes, and some cancers—especially colon cancer. Moreover, fiber can lower the risk for AMD.

What exactly is fiber? *Fiber*, which is found only in plants, is a type of carbohydrate that cannot be broken down by digestion and absorbed by the body. There are two types of fiber—soluble and insoluble.

Soluble fiber dissolves in water, forming a gel-like mass that is fermented by the friendly bacteria in the large intestine, forming *short-chain fatty acids*. These short-chain fatty acids have only two to six carbon atoms (unlike essential fatty acids, which have at least eighteen carbon atoms). They act as an important food source for the cells that line your large intestine. Keeping the lining of your intestines well-fed is critical to your ability to absorb all the healthy nutrients provided by your diet. As you may already know, the gel formed by soluble fiber also bulks up your stools and guards against both constipation and diarrhea. In fact, a majority of the fiber supplements you'll find on the shelves of your local drugstore contain mostly soluble fiber.

Soluble fiber performs other important functions as well. It helps to lower LDL (low-density lipoprotein) or "bad" cholesterol, by trapping dietary cholesterol and fats and aiding in their elimination. Just as vital, it helps to increase your HDL (high-density lipoprotein) or "good" cholesterol. Soluble fiber also slows the body's absorption of dietary sugars, thereby helping to regulate blood glucose levels. All of these benefits make this form of fiber a great way to avoid heart disease, type 2 diabetes, and several other common disorders. Foods rich in soluble fiber include oatmeal, many fruits and vegetables—especially oranges, apples, blueberries, and carrots—beans, and barley. Be aware that most foods contain both soluble and insoluble fiber, but usually, a food is richer in one type than it is in the other.

Insoluble fiber does not dissolve in water, but adds bulk to your stools and helps keep waste products moving along your digestive tract. This helps keep you regular. The more insoluble fiber you consume, the larger the stools. This kind of fiber pretty much passes unchanged from your body. However, scientists now think that insoluble fiber produces a small amount of fermentation, creating the short-chain fatty acids that we discussed above. Insoluble fiber also helps you to lose weight because the bulk makes you feel full and satisfied. Foods rich in insoluble fiber include wheat bran; most beans; lentils; flax seeds; vegetables such as okra, turnips, and peas; and many fruits (be sure to include the skin). Eating an apple provides both types of fiber—soluble fiber on the inside of the apple and insoluble in the skin. When making a salad, add cabbage, onions, and peppers to the dark leafy greens to add extra insoluble fiber. A good high-fiber cereal will also increase your insoluble fiber intake. Just add some berries and a little milk, and you are all set!

What about fiber and AMD? Two studies suggest that consuming fiber-rich foods may decrease your risk for AMD. In one study, researchers reported that people in their forties to sixties who consumed fiber-rich vegetables four to seven times a week had a markedly *decreased* risk for drusen—the yellow fatty deposits that form under the retina—compared with people who consumed less fiber. In a second study, an Asian diet high in vegetables, legumes, fruit, whole grains, tomatoes, and seafood decreased the risk of AMD compared with a typical American diet, which contains much less fiber. So your grandmother was right about eating more roughage!

How Much Fiber Should You Consume Each Day?

Now you know why it's so important to include plenty of fiber in your diet. If you are like the average American, you are getting about 15 grams a day. That is not enough. The total daily dietary fiber intake for those over fifty years of age should be about 21 grams for women and 30 grams for men. We suggest that you gradually increase your fiber intake over a few weeks. If you increase it suddenly, you could get gas, abdominal bloating, cramping, and even constipation. Be sure to drink plenty of water to soften your stools. Aim for about eight cups of fluids each day. Choose foods from Table 9.1 to increase your intake of both soluble and insoluble fiber.

Table 9.1. Fiber-Rich Foods

Food Category	Food	Total Fiber
Fruits	Raspberries, 1 cup	8.0 g
	Apple with skin, 1 medium	4.4 g
	Banana, 1 medium	3.1 g
	Orange, 1 medium	3.1 g
	Strawberries, 1 cup	3.0 g
Grains, Cereal, and Pasta	Whole wheat spaghetti, cooked, 1 cup	6.3 g
	Bran flakes, $1/4$ cup	5.5 g
	Oatmeal, cooked, 1 cup	4.0 g
	Popcorn, air-popped, 3 cups	3.6 g
	Whole wheat bread, 1 slice	1.9 g
Legumes, Nuts, and Seeds	Split peas, boiled, 1 cup	16.3 g
	Black beans, boiled, 1 cup	15.0 g
	Lima beans, boiled, 1 cup	13.2 g
	Almonds, 1 ounce (23 nuts)	3.5 g
	Pecans, 1 ounce (19 halves)	2.7 g
Vegetables	Green peas, boiled, 1 cup	8.8 g
	Broccoli, boiled, 1 cup	5.1 g
	Sweet corn, boiled, 1 cup	3.6 g
	White potato with skin, baked, 1 small	2.9 g
	Tomato paste, canned, $1/4$ cup	2.7 g
	Carrot, 1 raw	1.7 g

■ PROTEIN

When you eat foods containing protein, your digestive juices break it down into smaller units called *amino acids;* in fact, amino acids are referred to as the "building blocks" of protein. All amino acids contain carbon, hydrogen, oxygen, and nitrogen atoms. There are nine *essential amino acids* that your body can't make, so you must get them from your diet. There are six other amino acids that you need to get from your diet during certain disease conditions, and five amino acids that can be synthesized by your body.

Your amazing body uses these twenty amino acids to build thousands of new proteins needed by all your cells, tissues, and organs. These proteins are very different from one another—with different structures, different combinations of amino acids, and different functions—but each depends upon having the right amino acids, or building blocks, available. You can see why it's crucial to get enough protein and essential amino acids.

When you think of protein sources, you may automatically think of meat as a good source, and it is. However, as you learned in the previous chapter, meat sources often come with too much saturated fats and cholesterol. Below, we'll talk about getting your protein from other sources.

Because of the importance of consuming proteins that provide all the essential amino acids, dietary proteins are divided into two groups according to the amino acids they contain. *Complete proteins,* which constitute the first group, contain ample amounts of all the essential amino acids. These proteins are found in meat, fish, poultry, cheese, eggs, milk, the grain quinoa (pronounced *keen-wah*), and soy. *Incomplete proteins,* which constitute the second group, offer only some of the essential amino acids. These proteins are found in foods such as grains, legumes, and leafy green vegetables.

Although it is important to maintain the full range of amino acids—both essential and nonessential—it is not necessary to get them from meat, fish, poultry, and the other complete-protein foods. It is possible to create complete proteins by combining the right incomplete-protein foods. This is called *food combining.* For instance, although beans and rice are individually quite rich in protein, each lacks one or more essential amino acids. However, when you combine beans and rice with each other, or when you combine either one with any of a number of other protein-rich foods, you form a complete protein that is a high-quality substitute for meat.

As you read in the last chapter, the specific proteins you eat affect your risk for AMD. Australian studies evaluated the effect of red meat versus chicken in more than 6,700 people age fifty-eight to sixty-nine. A high intake of red meat was associated with early AMD, while the consumption of chicken more than three and a half times a week was inversely associated with late AMD—the more chicken, the less late AMD, and vice versa. Another study compared the effects of Asian diets versus Western diets on the development of age-related macular degeneration. Asian diets, which are rich in seafood and plant sources of protein, decreased the risk of AMD, while Western diets, which are higher in red meat and lower in plants, were associated with the progression of early AMD to late AMD. So choosing poultry and seafood over meat and adding more plant protein to your diet can be quite helpful to your eyes and your overall health.

How Much Protein Should You Consume Each Day?

To calculate your protein needs, take your weight in pounds and multiply it by 0.36 to get the minimal number of grams of protein you should consume each day. This amounts to about 56 grams, or 2 ounces, for the average sedentary man, and 46 grams, or 1.5 ounces, for the average sedentary woman. This is the *minimum* amount of protein you need to consume. For example, a sedentary women weighing 140 pounds might eat one egg (6 g), six ounces of yogurt (17 g), a glass of low-fat milk (8 g), and three ounces of salmon (21 g), for a total of 52 g. She could well consume more without risking serious health problems such as mood disorders, digestive problems, and kidney problems, which occur when a person's diet is over-loaded with excessive protein!

How much protein is too much? Instead of multiplying your weight by 0.36, multiply it by 1.1. So our 140-pound lady could safely eat double—theoretically, even triple—the amount calculated above. But she'll want to leave room in her diet for other healthy foods. Use the information presented in Table 9.2 to choose foods that will help you meet your protein requirements without getting an excess amount of this nutrient.

Table 9.2. Protein-Rich Foods

Food	Serving Size	Protein
Round steak	3 ounces	23 g
Tuna, salmon, trout, etc.	3 ounces	21 g
Turkey or chicken	3 ounces	19 g
Greek yogurt	6 ounces	17 g
Cottage cheese	1/2 cup	14 g
Cooked beans	1/2 cup	8 g
Milk	1 cup	8 g
Quinoa	1 cup	8 g
Tofu	4 ounces	10 g
Cooked whole wheat pasta	1 cup	7 g
Nuts	1/4 cup	7 g
Eggs	1 egg	6 g

■ GOOD FATS

In Chapter 7, we discussed the benefits of essential fatty acids (EFAs)—special fats that your body needs to form cell membranes, for their antioxidant and anti-inflammatory properties, and for much more. Included in the discussion was the importance of EFAs to eye health, as well as guidelines for taking EFAs in the form of supplements as a means of preventing or treating AMD. (See the discussion of EFAs, which begins on page 95, and the table of supplements, which begins on page 101.) But even if you're taking EPA/DHA supplements as recommended in that chapter, it is important to include EFAs in your diet, because foods rich in fatty acids offer many other valuable nutrients that work with the EFAs. You usually don't get that in supplements.

As you may remember, there are two families of essential fatty acids—omega-3s and omega-6s. Both are necessary for life, but most Americans don't get enough omega-3 fatty acids and consume too many omega-6s. In Chapter 7, you learned about EPA (eicosapentae-noic acid) and DHA (docosahexaenoic acid), two omega-3 fatty acids found in some fish. Another important omega-3 is ALA (alpha-lino-lenic acid), which is found in some plants and plant oils. The major omega-6 fatty acid supplied by your diet, LA (linoleic acid), is found in many different foods.

Food sources of the omega-3 fatty acids EPA and DHA include fatty fish such as herring, mackerel, and salmon. Plant sources of the omega-3 fatty acid ALA include flaxseed and its oil; walnuts and their oil; canola oil; some beans, including navy, northern, and pinto; and dark green leafy vegetables. Some eggs contain small amounts of ome-ga-3s because the chickens are given feed that's high in omega-3s.

Food sources of omega-6 fatty acids include vegetable oils, such as corn, soy, safflower, and sunflower oils; plus most nuts and seeds, such as sesame seeds, Brazil nuts, pecans, pumpkin seeds, peanuts, and almonds. Commercial salad dressings, mayonnaise, margarine, cookies and cakes, and many other processed foods are also full of omega-6 fatty acids because they are prepared with the omega-6-rich oils mentioned above. Fatty meats and poultry also include omega-6s.

How Much "Good Fat" Should You Consume Each Day?

In Chapter 7 (see Table 7.1), we recommend a daily supplement of EPA and DHA omega-3 fatty acids. When it comes to the foods you put on your plate, we advise you to include all of the sources of omega-3 fatty acids. Enjoy ground flaxseeds, walnuts, walnut oil, and dark green leafy vegetables such as kale and spinach, which are all good sources of ALA; and eat at least two servings a week (three ounces each) of fatty fish such as herring, sardines, salmon, and tuna, which supply EPA and DHA. (When consuming oils, nuts, and seeds, stick to the number of servings recommended in Table 10.3, which starts on page 184.)

What about omega-6 fatty acids? As already mentioned, most people in Western society consume too many omega-6s. Certainly, it's healthy to have reasonable amounts of Brazil nuts, pecans, pump-kin seeds, and the other nuts and seeds that contain omega-6s. But you'll want to replace corn oil and other oils rich in omega-6s with oils that offer omega-3s; and you'll want to entirely avoid highly processed foods, which are full of the "anti-nutrients" that increase the risk of AMD.

Table 9.3 enables you to quickly recognize food sources of both omega-3 and omega-6 fatty acids.

Table 9.3. Essential Fatty Acid-Rich Foods

Food	Serving Size	Omega-6 Fatty Acids	Omega-3 Fatty Acids		
		LA	ALA	EPA	DHA
Canola oil	1 tablespoon		1.3 g		
Flaxseed oil	1 tablespoon		7.3 g		
Walnut oil	1 tablespoon		1.4 g		
Corn oil	1 tablespoon	7.3 g			
Soybean oil	1 tablespoon	6.9 g	0.9 g		
Kidney beans	3 ounces	0.1 g	0.2 g		
Pecans, roasted in oil	1 ounce	6.4 g			
Kale, raw	1 cup		0.1 g		
Spinach, raw	1 cup		.04 g		
Walnuts, English	1 ounce		2.6 g		
Herring, Pacific	3 ounces			1.1 g	0.8 g
Salmon, Chinook	3 ounces			0.9 g	0.6 g
Tuna, fresh, Yellowfin	3 ounces			0.2 g	0.1 g
Tuna, canned, white meat	3 ounces			0.2 g	0.5 g
Tuna, canned, light meat	3 ounces			0.04 g	0.2 g

■ VITAMINS AND MINERALS

In earlier chapters, we discussed why certain vitamins and minerals are important for fighting AMD. Many of these nutrients are strong antioxidant and anti-inflammatory agents. Some are important for the control of blood sugar levels and cardiovascular health, and therefore indirectly protect your eyes. And many perform functions that directly contribute to eye health. (For details, see Chapter 7.)

Before the advent of nutritional supplements, people got their vitamins and minerals from the foods they ate. This was ideal because unlike manmade supplements, foods contain other nutrients that work in harmony with vitamins and minerals, helping the body absorb and use them. It's important to be aware, though, that our foods often offer fewer nutrients than they did years ago. The declining nutritional value of our food supply was studied by a team of researchers from the University of Texas. After examining the U.S. Department of Agriculture's nutritional data from both 1950 and 1999 for forty-three different fruits and vegetables, they reported significant reductions in protein, calcium, phosphorus, iron, vitamin B_2, and vitamin C. The researchers concluded that one of the main reasons for these declining levels was soil depletion. Crops are grown in soil that has been depleted of its nutrients by repeated farming. This means that this year's crops will contain fewer nutrients than last year's crops, and so on. The nutritional value of our crops has also been affected by the breeding of new plants that grow faster, grow larger, are more resistant to pests, survive dryness and heat, and provide the more intense flavors and sweetness that consumers have come to demand. Nutritional value is not usually one of the goals of commercial farmers.

Despite their findings regarding declining nutrient levels, the University of Texas researchers concluded, "Currently available vegetables and fruits are still our most broadly nutrient-dense foods, and hundreds of studies document their superior health-promoting qualities." We recommend that you both take supplements *and* choose healthy foods to insure that your "eye factory" is getting all the raw materials it needs for normal vision. Table 9.4 will guide you to the best food sources for a number of important nutrients.

Table 9.4. Sources of Vitamins and Minerals Important in AMD

Nutrient	Plant Sources	Animal Sources
VITAMINS		
Vitamin A		Fish and liver.
Beta-Carotene and other Carotenoids	Carrots, sweet potatoes, and dark leafy greens.	
Vitamin B_6 (Pyridoxine)	Potatoes, starchy vegetables, and non-citrus fruits.	Fish, beef, and beef liver.
Vitamin B_9 (Folate)	Fruits, vegetables, peas, beans, and nuts.	Beef liver and eggs.
Vitamin B_{12} (Cobalamin)		Fish, poultry, meat, eggs, and dairy.
Vitamin C	Oranges and other citrus fruits, red peppers, kale, Brussels sprouts, broccoli, and strawberries.	
Vitamin D		Fatty fish, beef liver, egg yolks, and vitamin D-fortified milk products.
Vitamin E	Olive oil, almonds and other nuts, seeds, green leafy vegetables, and wheat germ.	
MINERALS		
Chromium	Whole grains, brewer's yeast, bran cereal, Brazil nuts, orange juice, pears, tomatoes, romaine lettuce, onions, broccoli, potatoes, and green beans.	Shellfish and pork.
Copper	Nuts and seeds, legumes, cherries, avocados, and whole grains.	Liver, oysters, eggs, and poultry.
Magnesium	Dark green leafy vegetables, nuts and seeds, beans, whole grains, avocados, bananas, and dark chocolate.	Fish and yogurt.

Nutrient	Plant Sources	Animal Sources
MINERALS (cont.)		
Potassium	Avocado, spinach, sweet potatoes, dried apricots, white beans, bananas, and acorn squash.	
Zinc	Beans, nuts, whole grains, and fortified breakfast cereals.	Oysters, red meat, poultry, crab, lobster, milk, and cheese.

■ PHYTOCHEMICALS

Phytochemicals—literally, "plant chemicals"—are the natural biologically active compounds that give plants their distinctive tastes, colors, and aromas. Phytochemicals not only make foods like blueberries and carrots brightly colored and attractive, but also provide some very important nutrients. You'll find these compounds in fruits, vegetables, grains, beans, nuts, and plant-based beverages such as tea and wine. (Egg yolks also contain phytochemicals because the chickens that lay them consume corn, which contains yellow pigments.) These chemicals are not essential in the way that vitamins, minerals, and essential fatty acids are. Our bodies could perform without them; however, they protect our metabolic processes and cells from oxidative stress, defending us from cancer, heart disease, and age-related disorders like AMD. Choosing a variety of fruits and veggies in a rainbow of colors will insure that you get the phytochemicals that are vital for healthy eyes.

Carotenoids

Carotenoids are plant pigments responsible for the bright yellow, orange, and red colors of a number of fruits and vegetables, including butternut squash, cantaloupe, carrots, mangoes, nectarines, oranges, yellow peppers, pineapple, pumpkin, and more. In plants, these compounds absorb light energy for use in photosynthesis and protect the green pigment chlorophyll from being damaged by light. In human beings, these compounds have a range of protective functions.

There are so many carotenoids—over 700 are found in nature, with 60 or so found in foods—that it is useful to break them into categories.

Provitamin A Carotenoids

The *provitamin A carotenoids*—which include beta-carotene and several other compounds—are carotenoids that can be converted by the body into a type of active vitamin A called retinol. As you learned in Chapter 7, vitamin A is crucial to the maintenance of eye health. As a powerful antioxidant, it is involved in reducing inflammation and fighting free-radical damage, both of which contribute to AMD. It is also an integral part of the transformation of light energy into nerve impulses, a process that permits images to reach the brain. When you don't consume enough carotenoids, your eyes are more vulnerable to damage by sunlight, which increases your risk for AMD.

The provitamin A carotenoids are found in a wide range of fruits and vegetables, with some of the best sources being carrots, pumpkin, sweet potatoes, and butternut squash. (See Table 9.5 for a more complete list of foods.)

Lutein, Zeaxanthin, and Meso-Zeaxanthin

The three major carotenoids found in high concentrations in the macula are lutein, zeaxanthin, and meso-zeaxanthin. Lutein and zeaxanthin are both of dietary origin, while meso-zeaxanthin is derived from lutein. (Lutein is converted into meso-zeaxanthin in the retina.) As you learned in earlier chapters, long-term exposure to blue light is believed to increase the risk of AMD. These three carotenoids form the macular pigment, which prevents a substantial amount of the blue light from entering the eye and causing damage. Note that these nutrients are sometimes classified as *xanthophylls* or *nonprovitamin A carotenoids* because, unlike compounds such as beta-carotene, they are *not* converted into vitamin A in the body.

Recently, a group of Chinese scientists published a review of twenty studies that examined the effects which consuming either lutein, zeaxanthin, and meso-zeaxanthin *or* a placebo has on MPOD (macular pigment optical density). The scientists concluded that those taking the carotenoids had higher blood levels of the nutrients and higher MPOD. Since increased MPOD is associated with a lower risk for age-related macular degeneration, it is clear that including lutein and zeaxanthin in your diet is critical for normal eye health. If you have higher MPOD, you will see better, experience less glare, and enjoy better contrast sensitivity—the ability to see under low light conditions.

Although you should be taking an AREDS2 supplement, which contains lutein, it's important to also get lutein and zeaxanthin in your food, since the fruits and vegetables that are rich in these nutrients also provide other important nutrients. The best sources of lutein are dark green leafy vegetables like spinach, kale, turnip greens, and collard greens. Although lutein is found in plants, when animals eat plants, lutein is stored in their eggs and fat. For that reason, egg yolks are another good source of lutein. Good sources of zeaxanthin include orange bell peppers, orange juice, yellow corn, honeydew melon, mangoes, and kiwi fruit.

Lycopene

Lycopene is another member of the carotenoid family. Of all the carotenoids, lycopene is the most potent antioxidant, which means that it is especially effective at neutralizing the free radicals that are so destructive to cells and their membranes. According to the American Cancer Society, the antioxidant activity of lycopene is at least twice as great as that of beta-carotene. Considering lycopene's antioxidant capability, it should come as no surprise that, as reported in the *Archives of Ophthalmology,* people who have the lowest serum levels of lycopene are twice as likely to have age-related macular degeneration compared with people who have the highest serum levels of lycopene.

Lycopene is found in red fruits and vegetables, including tomatoes, watermelon, pink grapefruit, apricots, pink guava, and papaya. Usually, to get the greatest nutritional benefit from fruits and vegetables, it's best to eat them whole and unprocessed. This is not true of lycopene, which is better absorbed from processed tomato products. So while you'll get some lycopene—as well as other important nutrients—from a bowl of watermelon chunks or half of a pink grapefruit, you'll get a bigger boost of this nutrient from canned tomato purée, canned tomato juice, or canned vegetable juice cocktail. If high salt content is a problem for you, be sure to look for low-sodium tomato products.

Flavonoids

Flavonoids are a large group of phytochemicals—with over 6,000 members—that add flavor and color to fruits and vegetables. These nutrients are important in preventing and treating eye disease because of their strong antioxidant effects. They convert highly reactive free radicals to less reactive free radicals, they inhibit certain enzymes involved in generating free radicals, and they can inactivate metals that may produce free radicals. Flavonoids are also important because they increase blood flow in the eye and help prevent leakage in the retina. Finally, flavonoids have an anti-inflammatory effect.

Fruits that are high in flavonoids include blueberries and other berries, bananas, and citrus fruits. Flavonoid-rich vegetables include parsley, onions, sweet potatoes, romaine lettuce, and tomatoes. Black and green teas are also good sources of these phytochemicals, as is dark chocolate. Although studies have not yet shown that cocoa has a direct effect on AMD, in one preliminary study, consumption of cocoa flavonoids improved visual function in young adults. Cocoa has also been shown to reduce inflammation, increase HDL cholesterol, and have other effects that have been associated with a reduced risk of AMD. Just be sure to choose a cocoa product that's high in cocoa and low in sugar. (See the discussion on page 73.)

Anthocyanins are the most prominent members of the flavonoid family. Known for their anti-inflammatory properties, they are associated with lower risks of hypertension, cancer, and cognitive decline, and they have been shown to prevent blood vessel damage, which is part of the wet AMD disease process. Anthocyanins have also been linked to better visual acuity. Tests suggest that these phytochemicals may improve overall vision and be especially beneficial for night vision. In one study, taking bilberry and black currant anthocyanin supplements temporarily enhanced the vision of thirty-six patients. As yet, there have been no specific studies of the effect of anthocyanins on AMD, but there is evidence that consuming more fruits in

Table 9.5. Eye-Protecting Phytochemicals and Their Sources

Phytochemical	Food Source	Other Benefits of These Foods
Provitamin A Carotenoids (such as beta-carotene)	Orange and yellow fruits and vegetables such as yellow apples, apricots, butternut squash, cantaloupe, carrots, mangoes, nectarines, oranges, papayas, peaches, pears, yellow bell peppers, persimmons, pineapple, pumpkin, rutabagas, yellow summer or winter squash, sweet potatoes, and lemons.	Many of the fruits and vegetables rich in these carotenoids also contain vitamin C, omega-3 fatty acids, folate (B_9), and fiber.
Lutein and Zeaxanthin	Broccoli; red, orange, and yellow bell peppers; carrots; collard greens; yellow corn; honeydew melons; kale; oranges and orange juice; spinach; tomatoes; and red spices such as cayenne pepper and paprika. Because chickens eat corn, lutein is also found in egg yolks.	Leafy greens such as spinach and kale are also good sources of folate (B_9), vitamin K, potassium, omega-3 fatty acids, and fiber.
Lycopene	Red and orange fruits and vegetables such as apricots, guavas, watermelon, tomatoes, processed tomato products such as tomato paste, papaya, pink grapefruit, and red bell peppers.	Many red fruits are also high in vitamin C and folate (B_9).
Flavonoids (such as anthocyanins)	Cocoa; bananas; dark beans, such as black and kidney beans; berries; nuts; onions; parsley; romaine lettuce; sweet potatoes; tomatoes; tree fruits, such as bananas, citrus fruits, apples, pears, plums, and peaches; and black and green tea. For anthocyanins, choose red-orange and blue-violet produce such as berries, eggplant, plums, and prunes.	Many red fruits are also high in vitamin C and folate (B_9). A number of these fruits and vegetables also include fiber.

general lowers the risks for AMD. And, as you've seen, these nutrients appear to offer benefits to the eyes.

Varying amounts of anthocyanins are found in fruits and vegetables that have red-orange to blue-violet colors. To maximize your consumption of anthocyanins, choose the most vibrantly colored produce you can find. Red Delicious and Gala apples provide more anthocyanins than Fuji or green apples, while black raspberries are a richer source than red raspberries. Concord grapes have more of these nutrients than red grapes, which have more than green grapes. Other produce that's rich in anthocyanins includes eggplant, chokeberries, blackberries, and elderberries.

CONCLUSION

Now you know which dietary components—fiber, protein, essential fatty acids, vitamins and minerals, and phytochemicals—can support eye health and help prevent or slow the progress of age-related macular degeneration. Throughout this chapter, we have mentioned many of the foods that provide these important nutrients. If you're wondering how you will take all of this information and turn it into an effective Anti-AMD Diet, you need wonder no more. In the next chapter, we will explain how you can choose healthy foods and create a delicious diet that will not only safeguard your eyes but also help prevent a range of serious disorders, from diabetes to heart disease.

10

Choosing Foods to Put on Your Plate

In Chapter 9, you learned about the nutritional components that are especially important for eye health—fiber, protein, essential fatty acids, vitamins and minerals, and phytochemicals. Now comes the fun part! We'll help you choose all the delicious foods that can provide these components—fruits and vegetables, whole grains, poultry, fish, meat, nuts, beans and lentils, low-fat dairy products, and more. We've even included a discussion of safe sweeteners, which you can use in place of refined sugar and artificial sweeteners.

Eating for eye health doesn't have to be complicated or difficult. This chapter will show you how to select the best foods for your Anti-AMD Diet. We'll look at each group of foods separately, but for an overview of your new diet, simply turn to Table 10.3 on page 184.

FRUITS AND VEGETABLES

Researchers have long believed that consuming at least five servings of fruits and vegetables each day reduces your risk for age-related diseases. But a new study from London reported even better results when participants consumed *ten servings a day*. These researchers studied some 2 million people—a very large sample for a scientific study—by condensing 95 studies into one. They found that ten daily servings of fruits and vegetables significantly reduce the risks for heart disease (24 percent), stroke (33 percent), cardiovascular disease (28 percent), total cancer (13 percent), and premature death (31 percent). Dr. Dagfinn Aune, the lead author of the study, commented that there is no way to put the vast array of beneficial compounds into a pill. He said, "Most likely it is the whole package of beneficial nutrients you obtain by eating fruits and vegetables that is crucial to health. This is why it is important to eat whole plant foods to get the benefits."

Several studies have specifically examined the impact of a high intake of produce on patients with AMD. For example, a Harvard Medical School study examined the effects of the Mediterranean Diet, which is high in fruits, vegetables, whole grains, and fish, and low in red meat. It was found that a greater adherence to the Mediterranean diet decreased the risk of AMD progressing to advanced stages of the disease. Another study concluded that a high intake of fruit was protective against progression to late AMD.

As you know from Chapter 9, fruits and veggies provide you with lots of fiber, vitamins and minerals, some omega-3 essential fatty acids, and a wealth of different phytochemicals—those colored pigments that also influence the flavor and taste of plants. Any brightly colored fruit or vegetable provides antioxidants that tame the free radicals in your body, helping to prevent the damage that can lead to disorders such as age-related macular degeneration.

Each fruit or vegetable contains a unique set of nutrients. Let's look first at fruits, and then at vegetables. (To learn about the functions of specific nutrients, see Chapter 7. To learn about the function of dietary components such as fiber and essential fatty acids, see Chapter 9.)

■ FRUITS

Fruits are naturally low in fat, sodium, and calories, and are entirely free of cholesterol. They supply many essential nutrients that are under-consumed in the United States and other Western countries, including potassium, dietary fiber, vitamin C, vitamin A, and folic acid. As you learned in Chapters 7 and 9, these nutrients are necessary both for overall health and for the healthy functioning of your eyes.

Below, we've highlighted the important nutrients found in several different types of fruit. Please keep in mind that you should be eating the whole fruit—not just the juice. Although fruit juice provides a bounty of vitamins and minerals, the removal of fiber creates concentrated amounts of sugar that cause a rapid rise in blood glucose levels as soon as the juice is consumed. That is why you should always choose a whole apple over apple juice and a handful of grapes over a super-sweet glass of grape juice. Because of the fiber, fresh whole fruit also makes you feel more satisfied than a beverage. Turn to Table 10.3 to learn recommended portion sizes.

Citrus Fruits

Citrus fruits include oranges, grapefruit, tangerines, lemons, and limes These juicy treats supply vitamin C, folate, calcium, and potassium. Citrus fruits are also a rich source of phytochemicals—namely the flavonoids, which give these fruits their color and flavor. As you may remember from the previous chapter, flavonoids act as strong antioxidants and anti-inflammatory substances. The white pith of the fruit, found inside the skin, is an especially good source of flavonoids, so when peeling the fruit, try to leave some of the pith intact. If you doubt that whole fruit is better than juice, consider this: A whole orange provides five times more flavonoids than an eight-ounce glass of orange juice.

Berries

Blackberries, raspberries, blueberries, bilberries, loganberries, cranberries, and strawberries are all small bundles of healthy nutrients. They are rich sources of vitamin C and good sources of folic acid, as well as some potassium. As a bonus, all berries supply the fiber your body needs.

In Chapter 9, you learned about the most prominent member of the flavonoid family, the anthocyanins. Berries are also packed with these phytochemicals, which are known for their anti-inflammatory properties and their ability to fight disease—including heart disease, which is a risk factor for age-related macular degeneration.

Anthocyanins are responsible for the blue, black, and red colors of berries, so to be sure you're getting anthocyanin-rich fruit, choose the darkest colored berries you can find.

Considering the powerful nutrients found in berries, it should come as no surprise that studies often specifically mention the disease-fighting properties of these fruits. In a review paper published in the *Journal of Diabetes Investigation,* scientists concluded, "A higher intake of fruit, especially berries, and green leafy vegetables, yellow vegetables, cruciferous vegetables or their fiber is associated with a lower risk of type-2 diabetes." Other studies have looked at the effect of berries on AMD. In one study, human retinal cells in cell cultures were damaged with blue light. Cranberry extract was found quite effective in protecting the retinal cells from the blue light, and even helped them regenerate. In fact, cranberries are sometimes referred to as a superfruit because of their nutritional properties. They are rich in vitamins and minerals and dietary fiber, and contain an amazing array of potent phytochemicals, including flavonoids and phenolics. As you may know, because of the sourness of cranberries, cranberry juice and sauce are usually loaded with sugar or high-fructose corn syrup. As a healthy alternative, buy dried, unsweetened cranberries online, and add them to salads or yogurt, and make your own cranberry sauce, sweetening it with one of the healthier products discussed on page 177.

Melons

Watermelon, cantaloupe, honeydew, and casaba are rich sources of eye-healthy nutrients. For example, watermelon provides both vitamin A (in the form of beta-carotene) and vitamin C, as well as some potassium and the carotenoids known as lycopene, lutein, and zeaxanthin. Cantaloupe is thought to be one of the highest fruit sources of vitamin A (also in the form of carotenoids), plus potassium and small amounts of the B vitamins, including folate. While melon isn't the top fruit source of fiber, it does provide a portion of this necessary dietary component. A combination of different melon balls served in a pretty dish make a healthy, satisfyingly sweet dessert.

Peaches, Plums, Apricots, Nectarines, and Cherries

Sometimes called *stone fruits* or *drupes*, peaches, plums, apricots, nec-tarines, and cherries are synonymous with summer. Is there anything tastier than a peach enjoyed at its peak in summertime? Fortunately, stone fruits are also loaded with nutrients. All of them are good sources of vitamin C, potassium, and fiber, and many provide other nutrients, as well. Nectarines are a rich source of beta-carotene, for instance, while sweet cherries are rich in anthocyanins and other phytochemicals, carot-enoids such as lutein and zeaxanthin, and melatonin.

When shopping for these luscious fruits, be sure to pick varieties that are vividly colored, and are therefore packed with phytochemi-cals. Avoid peaches and nectarines with white flesh, and choose deep red cherries rather than pale ones. During the winter, when these fruits are not available in the produce section, consider using frozen fruit, which are generally picked at the peak of freshness and frozen within a few hours time. Just make sure that no sugar was added during processing.

Apples and Pears

Always available and relatively inexpensive, apples and pears are also good for you. Both fruits are rich in fiber: A medium apple pro-vides 4 grams of fiber, while a medium pear offers about 5 grams. They also provide potassium and vitamin C. Although they do not offer particularly high levels of other vitamins and minerals, apples and pears are rich in antioxidants such as polyphenols. Whenever possible, choose red apples and pears, as they also offer antho-cyanins, a powerful member of the flavonoid family. Be sure to eat the skin, as it contains a lion's share of the fruits' fiber and phytonu-trients. Skip the core, though, as the seeds of these fruits contain small amounts of cyanide.

Bananas and Plantains

Bananas are the world's most popular fruit! This is no surprise, as they are convenient to eat and truly delicious. Plantains are equally

161

tasty, although unlike bananas, they are usually cooked before you eat them.

Both bananas and plantains provide vitamin C, vitamin B_6, biotin, and essential minerals—potassium, magnesium, manganese, and copper. Plantains offer a generous amount of vitamin A, as well. As for fiber, a medium banana contains about 3 grams of fiber, including both soluble and insoluble fibers, and the same amount of plantain offers about 3.4 grams of fiber. Eating nuts or another protein source with a banana will help slow the absorption of all the natural sugar in bananas—about 14 grams, or 3.5 teaspoons. Green plantains have considerably less sugar than bananas.

Kiwi Fruits

Kiwi fruits are unique in two ways. First, their appearance—from their fuzzy skins to their seed-studded green flesh—is so striking and different from that of other fruits. Second, they have great nutrient density. Compared with other commonly consumed fruits, the kiwi is a powerhouse of nutrition because it is exceptionally high in vitamins C, E, and K; the minerals folate and potassium; and fiber. The kiwi is also a rich source of phytochemicals—the carotenoids, including beta-carotene, lutein, and the xanthophylls; and flavonoids, including the anthocyanins. Add some kiwi fruit to your diet, and enjoy the rewards.

No one knows exactly why a high fruit intake seems to protect against AMD, nor do they know which fruits offer the most protection. But they do know that fruit helps safeguard us from a myriad of common disorders, including AMD. Your best bet is to choose a wide variety of fruits of many different colors, and to enjoy at least five servings each day. Fruit is a sane way to enjoy sweetness without refined sugar and other unhealthy additives.

■ VEGETABLES

Like fruits, most vegetables are naturally low in fat and calories and contain no cholesterol. Vegetables also provide a variety of essential nutrients—potassium, folate, vitamin A in the form of beta-carotene, vitamin C, vitamin K, and dietary fiber. Lastly, vegetables are a rich source of phytochemicals. Just think of the yellow in yellow squash, the orange in pumpkin and sweet potatoes, the green that masks the color of many yellow-orange carotenoids present in green leafy vegetables, the red in beets, and the purple in red cabbage. As you know, when produce is vividly colored, it's full of health-promoting phytochemicals. Let's look at some of the families of veggies and see what they can add to your diet. Turn to Table 10.3 to learn recommended portion sizes.

Dark Green Leafy Vegetables

This category includes kale, collard greens, turnip greens, Swiss chard, spinach, red and green leaf lettuce, and romaine. These greens are a major source of iron and calcium, although the oxalic acid in Swiss chard and spinach prevents the body from absorbing the calcium. They are also excellent sources of folate and are loaded with carotenoids, including beta-carotene, lutein, and zeaxanthin.

If your salads are usually composed of iceberg lettuce or other light-colored greens, exchange them for their darker counterparts. Start with romaine, and mix in other leafy greens of your choosing—the darker, the better. Even if salads aren't your favorite food, you can still enjoy the benefits of dark leafy greens. Steam them as sides, use them to top a turkey burger, or add them to sandwiches instead of iceberg lettuce. They can also be included in smoothies. Using a blender, just purée kale or spinach with low-fat milk or a milk substitute, and add some yogurt, some frozen unsweetened strawberries, and a half banana for sweetness. You won't even realize you're drinking your vegetables!

The Cruciferous Vegetables

The cruciferous family of vegetables is large and includes cabbage, broccoli, cauliflower, Brussels sprouts, kale, and many more nutritious veggies. Brown and yellow mustard seeds and horseradish also belong to this family. These vegetables are nutritional superstars. They contain vitamin A in the form of carotenoids; B vitamins, including folate; vitamins C, E, and K; the minerals magnesium, manganese, potassium, and zinc; fiber; and protein. They are particularly high in one type of phytochemical, glucosinolates, which researchers have been studying as anti-cancer agents. Red cabbage also contains anthocyanins, which are flavonoids with powerful anti-inflammatory properties. Include these vegetables often in your meals, eating them raw, steamed, or quickly stir-fried to maintain their nutrients.

White and Sweet Potatoes

Although potatoes have gotten a bad rap because so many of them are turned into French fries, hash browns, loaded potato skins, or greasy chips, the white potato is really quite nutritious. When baked or boiled and consumed with the skin, the potato is a very good source of vitamin B_6 and a good source of vitamin C, copper, folate, manganese, niacin, potassium, phosphorus, pantothenic acid, and dietary fiber. It may come as a surprise that a large baked potato also offers as much protein as a serving of cheddar cheese. Prepare your spud without sour cream or butter. Instead, add a dollop of vegetarian chili or perhaps some steamed vegetables for a nutritious meal. Be sure to eat the skin, because that's where most of the fiber and some of the nutrients are found. And don't hesitate to try purple potatoes and other vibrantly colored varieties, as the colors indicate the presence of eye-protecting antioxidants.

An even more nutritious choice than a white potato is its distant relative, the sweet potato. You are probably familiar with the orange sweet potato, but these veggies also come in red, yellow, and purple. The orange ones are so rich in beta-carotene that they provide more than 438 percent of the recommended daily amount of vitamin A. They also provide 37 percent of the vitamin C and 15 percent of the fiber recommended for daily consumption, and they are excellent sources of potassium and manganese. Carotenoids other than beta-carotene make sweet potatoes a rich source of antioxidants. Red and purple sweet potatoes are equally nutritious, and are also excellent sources of anthocyanins. All in all, sweet potatoes are a nutritional treasure! Just don't add gobs of butter, brown sugar, and marshmallows, which can turn a great food into a nutritional nightmare. Instead, serve your sweet potato with a dash of your favorite herb or spice. Cinnamon, for instance, provides great taste, a touch of sweetness, and some seriously healthy antioxidants.

The Onion Family

This nutritious and flavorful family includes onions, garlic, leeks, shallots, scallions, and chives. These vegetables provide decent amounts of several vitamins and minerals, including vitamin C, vitamin B_6, folate, potassium, and fiber. But the onion's health benefits are thought to be chiefly the result of their high content of sulfur compounds, which act as natural blood thinners, and their phytochemicals, which include the strong antioxidant quercetin. Use onions in your cooking to flavor your dishes without the addition of salt or sugar.

Carrots, Celery, and Parsley

Carrots, celery, and parsley are all members of a family of aromatic flowering plants. Carrots have long been promoted for their beneficial effects on vision. This makes sense considering that these crunchy vegetables contain carotenoids beta-carotene, lutein, and zeaxanthin, which are essential for eye health. Carrots are also a good source of fiber; vitamins C, K, B_6, and folate; the minerals potassium, iron, copper, and manganese; and antioxidants.

A good source of dietary fiber, celery provides a decent amount of vitamin K as well as vitamin A, vitamin C, and calcium. Celery also contains the phytochemical coumarins, which may help prevent cancer by enhancing the activity of white blood cells.

Parsley is a good source of vitamins A, C, E, and K and the minerals iron, magnesium, and potassium. Of course, this flavorful plant is usually eaten in small amounts, so we end up getting only small amounts of its nutrients.

Carrots and celery make great raw snacks, and along with parsley, they make flavorful additions to a range of cooked dishes. These three veggies can also be juiced together and enjoyed as a nutrient-packed beverage.

Beets

You might guess by looking at red beets and their juice that they have an immense quantity of phytochemicals, which give them their bright red color. They contain red betalain pigments, which display potent antioxidant and anti-inflammatory effects. Beets are also an excellent source of vitamins C and B_6; the minerals copper, folate, potassium, and manganese; and dietary fiber. Research has shown that beets can reduce hypertension and increase levels of nitric oxide. Nitric oxide is important because it dilates the blood vessels, increasing the blood flow in the heart and in the small vessels of the eye and retina. However, if you have wet AMD, it might be prudent to limit your intake of beets, because excessive nitric oxide may cause weak blood vessels to leak.

Be aware that not all beets are red. Golden beets, which have a yellow-orange color, are sweeter and less earthy tasting than red beets, and have a slightly different nutritional profile, but are just as healthy. Like red beets, they are high in fiber. They also provide vitamins A and C; the minerals potassium, calcium, and iron; plus lycopene, zeaxanthin, and flavonoids. In other words, they're packed with eye-healthy nutrients.

Beets are often used in salads, can be roasted for a delicious side dish, and are great juiced. If you choose to eat red beets, though, you may be startled by the sudden reddish color of your urine and feces a day or so afterwards. Don't worry: It's just that powerful red pigment.

Just as we don't know everything about fruits, there is still much to be learned about vegetables, including their effects on the development and progression of age-related macular degeneration. But right now, we do know that a diet which is high in veggies helps prevent serious disorders like heart disease and diabetes, which are risk factors for AMD. And we know that vegetables are packed with nutrients that have been shown to be beneficial for our eyes. This is ample reason to add a bounty of delicious vegetables to our diet every single day.

Would a completely plant-based diet slow the progression of AMD and give you a healthier life? This has not yet been studied in patients with AMD, but a plant-based diet seems to be quite helpful in controlling other age-related diseases. If you aren't ready to go completely vegan, you can still dramatically increase your servings of fruit and vegetables!

BEANS, PEAS, AND LENTILS

Collectively known as legumes, beans, peas, and lentils are true super foods. They are high in protein and also offer both soluble and insoluble fiber; B-complex vitamins, especially folate; essential minerals, including calcium, iron, magnesium, potassium, and zinc; and several phytonutrients. This mix of nutrients enables beans to decrease insulin levels, improve metabolic syndrome, lower cholesterol, reduce high blood pressure, and even decrease the rate of cancer progression. Although no studies have been done to examine the relationship between legumes and macular degeneration, it's easy to see that this food group helps control the disorders that are known to be risk factors for AMD.

It should be noted that although legumes are a good protein source, they do not contain all nine of the essential amino acids, and are therefore not complete proteins. However, if you combine them with whole grains such as brown rice, you will get all of the amino acids your body needs. Be aware that, contrary to what experts used to believe, you do not have to get all of the essential amino acids at one meal. As long as you consume them over the course of a day, the body is able to produce the protein it requires. In fact, whenever you digest protein, the body breaks it down into amino acids and then puts it back together again into the specific forms of protein needed.

Choose from among a wide range of legumes, including black beans, black-eyed peas, cannellini beans, chickpeas (garbanzo beans), edamame (soybeans), kidney beans, lentils, pinto beans, split peas, and more. Beans that you cook yourself are the healthiest choice, because you control the amount of sodium being used. They are also the most economical to use. If you prefer the convenience of canned beans, either choose lower-sodium brands or place the beans in a sieve and rinse them thoroughly under cold running water to wash away as much of the sodium as possible. (By rinsing and draining canned beans, you can eliminate up to 41 percent of the sodium.) Then use them in salads, soups, side dishes, and entrées. We recommend at least a half-cup of beans a day.

NUTS

Nuts are high in protein, high in fiber, rich in essential fatty acids, and also offer nutrients such as calcium, copper, magnesium, phosphorus, selenium, vitamin E, some B vitamins, beta-carotene, lutein, and zeaxanthin. Nuts are also antioxidant powerhouses. Walnuts are the highest in heart- and eye-healthy omega-3s, but all nuts boast impressive nutritional profiles, including almonds, Brazil nuts, cashews, hazelnuts, peanuts, pecans, pine nuts, pistachios, and more. These rich-tasting morsels have been found to lower cholesterol and triglycerides, decrease fasting blood sugar, and decrease chronic inflammation. Therefore, it is not surprising that a 2016 Norwegian study reported that the regular consumption of nuts—only a handful a day—is associated with reduced cardiovascular disease, cancer, and death from respiratory disease, diabetes, and infections.

Purchase nuts in raw, unsalted form, and store in a dry, cool place. Avoid roasted nuts, as high heat destroys some of the nuts' nutrients. Remember that 80 percent of a nut is fat, and even though this is mostly healthy fat, it means a lot of calories. That's why you should eat nuts in moderation. Enjoy a handful of nuts (about 1.5 ounces) up to four times a week, or have two tablespoons of nut butter, spreading it on whole wheat bread or a crisp stalk of celery. Be sure to purchase a nut butter that contains only nuts, with no added oil, salt, or sugar. Better yet, make you own nut butter by swirling the nuts of your choice in a blender.

WHOLE GRAINS

In Chapter 8, we talked about the importance of avoiding white flour and other foods that have been stripped of most of their nutrients by food manufacturers. In contrast, eating at least three servings per day of *whole* grains has been shown to significantly decrease the risks of age-related disease—heart disease by 25 to 36 percent, stroke by

37 percent, type 2 diabetes by 21 to 27 percent, some cancers, and obesity. Two studies mentioned earlier suggest that the Mediterranean Diet and the standard Asian diet, which include whole grains as part of a healthy eating plan, decrease the risk for AMD. Despite this important information, only *4 percent* of adult Americans are consuming at least three servings of whole grains daily!

Here's why it's so important to choose whole grains. Every whole grain kernel consists of three parts—the bran, endosperm, and germ—each of which contributes different nutrients. The bran, which is the outer layer or shell, provides fiber, antioxidants, B vitamins, phytochemicals, and a significant amount of minerals, including iron, copper, zinc, and magnesium. The endosperm, which is the middle layer of each kernel, contains starch, some protein, and small amounts of some B vitamins and minerals. The germ, which is the embryo located in the center of the kernel, contains healthy fatty acids, B vitamins, phytochemicals, and antioxidants like vitamin E. It's responsible for the growth of the seed into a plant. There are literally hundreds of different phytochemicals in whole grains. When grains are refined, the bran and germ are removed, and with those parts of the grain go most of the grain's nutrients. You can see why choosing whole grains can make a big difference to your health.

Many whole grains can be cooked and then enjoyed hot as a side dish or hot cereal, or cooled and used to make a nutritious salad. A partial list of these healthy grains includes amaranth, hulled or pearled barley, brown rice, bulgur wheat (cracked whole wheat), whole wheat couscous, farro, oats, quinoa, and wheat berries. More healthy options are finding their way to supermarket and health food store shelves all the time, so you're sure to find a few that you love.

Whenever you purchase a product that's based on grains—bread, crackers, pasta, and cold cereals, for instance—be certain that the package is marked "100 percent whole grain." If a package of bread or crackers lists "wheat flour" in its ingredient list, the product is not *whole* wheat. If the package says, "contains whole wheat," the product may contain mostly refined wheat and perhaps only one-percent whole wheat! Another common and misleading term is "multigrain." This sounds very healthy, but it simply means that the product contains more than one type of grain—wheat and oats, for instance. The grains are mostly likely refined unless the package specifies "whole grain." Manufacturers play these games to trick you into buying a nutritionally deficient product. Don't play along! There are lots of 100-percent whole grain products to choose from—breads, cereals, crackers, pasta, bagels, wraps, tortillas, and so on. Read the ingredients lists carefully so that you won't be fooled by misleading marketing terms.

You should be getting at least three servings of whole grains a day, and there are many different ways in which you can enjoy this satisfying food. A serving is equal to: $^1/_2$ cup cooked rice or other whole grain, 1 cup ready-to-eat cereal (watch out for added sugar!), $^1/_2$ cup cooked pasta,1 slice bread, 5 small whole wheat crackers, 2 pieces Ry-Krisp crisp bread, 1 small tortilla, or 3 cups popcorn (no butter or salt!). If you are consuming less than three servings daily, add more whole grains to your diet.

MEAT, POULTRY, SEAFOOD, EGGS, AND OTHER PROTEIN SOURCES

In Chapter 9, you learned about the body's need for protein. Although requirements depend on weight, men need about 56 grams of protein per day, and women, about 46 grams. As explained earlier in this chapter, your protein requirements can be satisfied by vegetables, legumes, and grains. Milk and milk products also contribute protein to the diet. But for many people, meat, poultry, and seafood are the chief sources of dietary protein, and the protein you choose can have a major effect on your overall health and the well-being of your eyes.

As you've already learned, your eye health is likely to be better if you select chicken more often than beef. A research study carried out by Dr. Elaine Chong and colleagues from Australia's University of Melbourne followed over 6,000 people for thirteen years. The study involved monitoring the diet of the subjects and also taking high-definition photos of the subjects' retinas. At the end of the study, it was found that those who ate red meat more than ten times a week had a 47-percent higher risk of getting AMD than those who ate it only five times a week. Moreover, people who ate white meat chicken between three and four times a week had a 60-perccent lower risk of getting

AMD than those who ate chicken less than twice a week. Considering that a high-meat diet has long been associated with heart disease and other serious health disorders, it makes sense to lower your intake of red meat (beef, pork, and lamb) and to enjoy more meals that include white meat chicken. To control cholesterol, saturated fat, and calories, choose lean cuts of meat and enjoy your chicken without the fatty skin. Avoid luncheon meats—highly processed meats such as hot dogs, ham, and most of the meats you find at a deli counter. These are likely to contain nitrites or nitrates, sugar or high fructose corn syrup, and a lot of fat and salt, all of which can be damaging to your health.

As you know, one of the best places to find eye-healthy omega-3 fatty acids, first discussed on page 95, is your local fish store. Look for salmon, sardines, albacore tuna, herring, mackerel, and other fatty fish. Cod, catfish, clams, scallops, and shrimp are also healthy choices, even though they are not great sources of omega-3s. To maintain the health benefits of your seafood, avoid deep frying it or adding heavy sauces. Instead, sauté it in a little olive oil, broil it, or bake it, and add a squeeze of lemon.

Another good source of protein is eggs. Moreover, the yolk is a rich source of lutein and zeaxanthin, which accumulate in the macular pigment of the retina, protecting it from the damage associated with age-related macular degeneration. If possible, buy eggs that were produced by hens fed an omega-3 enriched diet, as these provide five times as much omega-3s as conventional eggs. Ask your doctor how many eggs you can eat a week given your cholesterol levels, and as often as possible, prepare your eggs by poaching or soft-boiling rather than frying or scrambling. Prolonged heat oxidizes the cholesterol, starting a process that can lead to plaque formation in the blood vessels.

If you are a vegetarian or you want to avoid the fat and cholesterol found in meat and poultry, consider getting at least some of your protein from soybean-based foods like tofu and seitan. While there have been no studies of the effects of soy foods on AMD, they are considered a good protein alternative.

How much of these protein sources should actually be on your plate each day? We suggest that every day, you have up to six ounces of white meat poultry (two portions, three ounces each), or three ounces of poultry and three ounces of fish. (Note that a three-ounce portion is about the size of a deck of cards.) Enjoy a three-ounce serving of fish—preferably omega-3-rich fatty fish—two or three times a week. Because a diet high in red meat has been linked to an increased risk for AMD, we recommend limiting the consumption of red meat to one serving (three ounces) once or twice a week. If possible, buy organic products and choose grass-fed beef, which is higher in omega-3 fatty acids and antioxidant nutrients. Finally, one egg a day, preferably marked "omega-3" on the package, is considered not only safe, but truly healthy.

DAIRY PRODUCTS AND ALTERNATIVES

For several years now, there has been a controversy over milk and milk products. Some people claim that milk is meant only for babies, while others point out all of the valuable nutrients it contains. We believe that milk's impressive nutritional profile make it a valuable part of your diet. One cup of skim milk offers 8 grams of protein containing all the essential amino acids. If you are consuming a 2,000-calorie diet, that cup of milk provides only 86 calories, no saturated fat, 50 percent of your daily calcium needs, 20 percent of vitamin B_2, 16 percent of vitamin B_{12}, 25 percent of phosphorus, and 12 percent of potassium, with only a trace of saturated fat. Milk is also fortified with 115 IU of vitamin D. The regular consumption of low-fat dairy foods has been found to lower the risk for obesity, prediabetes, type 2 diabetes, hypertension, and heart disease, which are all risk factors for AMD. In fact, over a fifteen-year period, Australian researchers studied the relationship between dairy product consumption and the incidence of AMD. They divided the study group into fifths, depending on their dairy consumption. The study results showed that a lower consumption of dairy products (both regular and low-fat) was associated with an increased risk of developing late AMD. They also reported a significant association between a low intake of dairy products and problems with retinal blood vessels. The exact reason for this isn't clear, but whether it's the calcium, the vitamins and minerals, or some other factor, it's encouraging news for everyone who loves dairy. To maximize the benefits offered by dairy products and minimize health problems like allergies, choose non-GMO (non-genetically modified organism) dairy from grass-fed cows.

If you avoid milk because of allergies, lactose intolerance, or another issue, you'll find that most markets offer a good selection of nondairy milk substitutes, including soy milk, rice milk, almond milk, and coconut milk. When selecting a product for use, consider not just flavor but also the nutrients it has to offer. Table 10.1 shows selected nutrition facts for several types of milk, but be aware that different versions of the same nondairy milk can have different nutritional profiles, because some brands are fortified with vitamin D, calcium, or other nutrients to make them comparable to cow's milk. Also be aware that some milk alternatives are highly sweetened, which you'll want to avoid. If you choose a product that does not have all of the nutrients offered by dairy milk, be sure to get them from other foods in your diet.

Table 10.1. Key Nutrients in One Cup of Unsweetened Milk or Milk Substitute

Milk or Milk Substitute	Calories	Protein	Calcium	Vitamin D
Almond milk	37	1.0 g	481 mg	80 IU
Coconut milk	76	1.0 g	459 mg	80 IU
Cows' milk, skim	83	8.0 g	299 mg	120 IU
Rice milk	113	1.0 g	283 mg	101 IU
Soy milk	108	2.0 g	289 mg	80 IU

Yogurt is another dairy product that supplies many nutrients. One cup of plain low-fat yogurt has about 154 calories, 2.5 grams of saturated fat, and almost 13 grams of protein. It also provides about 45 percent of your daily calcium needs, 10 percent of magnesium, 35 percent of phosphorus, 16 percent of potassium, 15 percent of zinc, and 12 percent of selenium. It contains vitamin D only if the yogurt has been fortified, so read the label. As an added benefit, yogurt contains live cultures that offer a large number of health benefits. If you're looking for a higher amount of protein, choose a Greek-style yogurt, which can have over 20 g per cup. To avoid added sugar, always buy plain yogurt and sweeten with diced fruit or a little unprocessed honey. (See page 177.) Again, all nutrient values vary according to brand, so it's important to check each product's Nutrition Facts label.

Some dairy products—cheese, sour cream, and cream cheese, for instance—are very high in saturated fat, and should be eaten only rarely, and then, in modest amounts. Cream cheese, sour cream, heavy or whipping cream, half and half, and buttermilk are especially poor choices because they provide little calcium and protein and lots of saturated fats.

Try to eat two servings of low-fat dairy products a day. A serving is equivalent to 1 cup of milk, 1 cup of yogurt, or $1^1/_2$ ounces of low-fat cheese.

What about butter? Butter is made from animal fat, so it contains saturated fat. And as you learned in Chapter 8, high levels of saturated fat have been shown to be a risk factor for AMD. Margarine, on the other hand, contains vegetable oils, so it should be healthier. Unfortunately, not all margarines are created equal. Some contain trans fats, which are considered more dangerous than saturated fats. If you opt for margarine, your best choice would be a "soft" margarine—not a hard stick—that contains no trans fats. To determine this, you'll have to look at both the Nutrition Facts label, which should list 0.0 g trans fats, and the ingredients list, which should include no fully or partially hydrogenated oils. If you have high cholesterol, ask your doctor if using a spread fortified with plant stanols would be a good idea, as these can help reduce cholesterol levels. If you *must* use butter for its unique taste, try whipped or light butter, which has half the fat and calories of regular butter. Whatever spread you choose, use it sparingly, spreading just a teaspoon on a piece of whole grain bread.

VEGETABLE OILS AND DRESSINGS

When purchasing oils for your cooking needs, it's important to choose those that will help support your eye health as well as your general well-being. We recommend canola, walnut, and olive oil.

Canola oil contains ALA omega-3 fatty acids and healthy mono-unsaturated fats. Because of its neutral flavor, it is a great oil for baking, but it can also be used for sautéing, roasting, and salad dressings. Just be aware that high-temperature cooking reduces canola oil's nutritional benefits.

Walnut oil, too, provides omega-3 fatty acids and is rich in phytonutrients and antioxidants. Unlike canola oil, walnut oil has a rich, nutty flavor that enhances the taste of foods. The downside is that it shouldn't be heated, so you'll want to use it only in salad dressings, to toss with pasta, or to flavor cooked vegetables, chicken, or fish.

Although olive oil does not contain omega-3 fatty acids, health experts agree that this natural oil provides important health benefits. It is rich in monounsaturated oleic acid, which has strong anti-inflammatory properties, contains large amounts of antioxidants, and offers modest amounts of vitamins E and K. Perhaps because of these nutrients, olive oil has been found to protect against heart disease via numerous mechanisms, and heart disease is a major risk factor for AMD. It has also been found to lower blood pressure, which may decrease the pressure in the tiny blood vessels in your eyes, protecting these vessels from damage. And it has been shown to help control blood sugar and insulin sensitivity. In fact, although more research is needed, this delicious oil appears to be helpful in the treatment of AMD. Olive oil is an important part of the Mediterranean Diet, which, as mentioned earlier in the chapter, has been found to decrease the likelihood that AMD will progress to advanced stages of the disease. It can be used in salad dressings, to roast foods, to sauté foods at low temperatures, and to flavor cooked vegetables, fish, and chicken. Most people find the taste of olive oil too pronounced for baking.

For the greatest health benefits, always choose high-quality cold-pressed oils, which have been extracted without the use of chemicals, and select only extra-virgin olive oil. Purchase organic products if you can, especially when buying canola oil, which can contain GMOs. All oils are high in calories, so limit yourself to one or two tablespoons a day.

We urge you to make your own salad dressings using one of the oils recommended above and a good-quality wine or balsamic

Measuring the Antioxidant Capacity of Foods

Throughout Part Three of this book, we recommend foods that are high in *antioxidants*—substances such as beta-carotene that can quench free radicals, thereby preventing the cellular damage that contributes to disorders such as age-related macular degeneration. But looking at a list of antioxidants can tell you only so much about the free radical-fighting potential of a food. That's why researchers at the National Institutes of Health decided to create ORAC (Oxygen Radical Absorbance Capacity), which measures the effectiveness of the combination of antioxidants in a given food at incapacitating a particular free radical. In other words, instead of measuring the levels of specific nutrients—only some of which have been identified by scientists—ORAC measures the antioxidant *activity* of a food. Depending on the food's antioxidant power, it is given an ORAC score. The higher the score, the greater the antioxidant action. For instance, the score for antioxidant-packed walnuts is 13,541. The score for iceberg lettuce, which is far lower in nutrients, is about 406.

Table 10.2 (page 177) presents the ORAC scores of a few high-antioxidant foods according to the USDA Database for the Oxygen Radical Absorbance Capacity (http://www.orac-info-portal.de/download/ORAC_R2.pdf). Keep in mind that the score for each food is based on 100 grams, or about 3.5 ounces. That's why the scores for the spices seem astronomically high. But while you would never eat 100 grams of ground cloves at a meal, it's true that spices deliver a high concentration of antioxidants, making them a valuable addition to your meals. (See the discussion of herbs and spices on page 182.) Don't hesitate to visit the USDA website to find the ORAC scores of foods that are of interest to you.

Before you decide to choose foods based solely on the ORAC scale, remember that this is only part of the picture of a healthy diet. Many essential nutrients—protein and fiber, for instance—are *not* reflected by ORAC. So every day, it makes sense to include a wide variety of healthy foods in your meals, as this will help you get all the nutrients you need, including antioxidants.

vinegar. Olive and walnut oil are especially suitable for dressings, as they lend a delicious flavor to any salad. Try to avoid commercial dressings, most of which contain sugar, corn syrup, or other ingredients that you want to avoid. If you must buy a commercial dressing, look for one made with canola, walnut, or olive oil and no sweeteners. Organic products are usually your best bet, but always check the ingredients.

Table 10.2. ORAC Scores for Selected Foods

Food (100 g or 3.5 ounces)	ORAC	Food (100 g or 3.5 ounces)	ORAC
Cloves, ground	290,283	Apples, Red Delicious (with skin)	4,275
Cinnamon, ground	131,420	Cherries	3,747
Turmeric, ground	127,068	Goji Berries	3,290
Dark chocolate	20,823	Peanuts	3,166
Walnuts	13,541	Cabbage, red	3,145
Kidney beans	8,606	Lettuce, red leaf	2,426
Blackberries	5,905	Spinach	1,513
Raspberries	5,065	Broccoli	1,510
Blueberries	4,669	Multigrain bread (with whole grains)	1,421
Strawberries	4,302		

SWEETENERS

In Chapter 8, we explained that sugar—in all its many forms—is highly damaging to your health. We also discussed how artificial sweeteners, although noncaloric, have their own adverse effects on the body. And we pointed out that *all* sweeteners are addictive and stimulate your brain to want even more sugary sweetness as well as more food than your body actually requires.

We urge you to avoid sweetened commercial foods, like cookies, sweetened beverages, and sweetened cereals. But we know that sometimes, perhaps when you're baking or drinking a cup of tea or coffee, you may want to add a little sweetness. In those cases, we recommend that you use the following products, which have been found to be safer and better for you than refined sugar, corn syrup, and the like. Even when adding these sweeteners, we urge you to use the smallest amount possible. Your eyes will thank you!

Stevia

Stevia is a natural sweetener that comes from the leaves of a plant bearing the same name. It has been used for over 1,500 years to sweeten teas and medicines, especially in South America. Stevia is 200 to 350 times sweeter than sugar, so only a little is needed, making it a zero-calorie product. Some people object to its slightly bitter or licorice taste, although others love it. We've found that it works best in citrus-flavored foods and beverages.

Besides being noncaloric, stevia has another important advantage over sugar: It does not increase blood sugar levels. In one study, diabetics who used stevia for sixty days were found to have significantly lower fasting blood glucose and lower glucose levels after meals than did a control group that did not use stevia. The stevia users' triglycerides and markers of other fats were also significantly decreased.

Stevia comes in several forms. Since many of these products contain fillers, you'll want to look for a product such as whole leaf liquid stevia or dried stevia leaves—something that's 100-percent stevia.

Monk Fruit Powder

Monk fruit powder is derived from a fruit that was first cultivated in China. The sweetener is made by crushing the fruit and collecting the juice, which is dried to create a powdered extract. Like stevia, monk fruit powder is many times sweeter than cane sugar, so that you'll need to use only a small amount. Also like stevia, it is noncaloric and will not affect blood glucose levels. Be sure to buy *pure* monk fruit powder. Avoid products that contain fillers or other sweeteners, like dextrose.

Xylitol

Xylitol is considered a "sugar alcohol," although it's really not a sugar or an alcohol! The xylitol you buy in the store or online is processed from birch or corn husk fibers to form xylose, which is processed into xylitol. This sweetener is not completely calorie-free, but has about 33 percent fewer calories than sugar. It also doesn't raise glucose like sugar does. Yet another bonus is that it has been found to reduce the occurrence of cavities by actively inhibiting the growth of the bacteria that cause tooth decay.

Unfortunately, xylitol can also have adverse effects. For some people, this sweetener causes diarrhea, gas, and bloating. The effect is often dose-related, so decrease your intake if you start having gastrointestinal problems. Be aware, too, that xylitol is poisonous for dogs. Don't let your four-legged friends anywhere near this sweetener, as it can cause liver failure and death. Cats, too, can be harmed by xylitol.

If you choose to try xylitol, you should be able to find the powder in most health food stores. Use a tiny amount at first, and if that does not bother you, increase the amount slowly until you achieve the desired degree of sweetness.

Unprocessed Honey

Unprocessed honey is another sweetener you can use in small amounts. Here, we're not talking about ordinary supermarket honey, which has been heated and filtered, removing most of the nutrients. We're referring to locally grown organic raw honey, which you should be able to find in health food stores or at farmers markets. Look for the least processed honey you can find so that the sweetener's natural vitamins, minerals, and antioxidants are intact. Whenever possible, buy a dark-colored honey, as this product will contain more antioxidants.

In general, studies have shown that raw honey is better for you than refined sugar. Honey causes less of an increase in blood glucose levels than sugar, and some studies indicate that it may even lower your fasting blood glucose levels if consumed regularly. As already

179

mentioned, it also provides valuable nutrients. But honey is about 80 percent sugar by weight, and actually provides more calories per teaspoon than sugar—although honey is sweeter, so you'll tend to use less of it. The bottom line is that this sweetener, like all sweeteners, should be used only in small amounts. Also be aware that you should never give honey to a child younger than a year of age, as an infant's undeveloped immune system cannot handle the spores that might be present.

CONDIMENTS

Condiments can add color, taste, and enjoyment to your meals. But if you choose the standard condiments you have probably been using for years, you'll also be adding a lot of salt, sugar, unhealthy fats, extra calories, and maybe even artificial colors. Now that you are a smart label reader, you can look at both the Nutrition Facts and the ingredients lists and avoid products that are too high in sodium or sugar, contain corn syrup, feature artificial colors and flavors, or contain other "anti-nutrients." Below, you'll find some tips to keep in mind as you shop for condiments.

Ketchup

Ketchup is made from tomatoes, vinegar, and spices—which are all healthy. But unfortunately, it also contains a lot of salt and sugar, and some brands include high-fructose corn syrup. The lycopene in the tomatoes is a strong antioxidant and also tames inflammation, so ketchup isn't all bad. Just look for brands that are lower in salt and sugar, and use only small amounts.

Relish

Relishes may seem innocent because they're packed with vegetables, but very often, they're also packed with corn syrup, sodium, and artificial colors—yellow and blue dyes that make the product appear greener. Opt for organic brands that omit the dyes, check the sugar and sodium counts, and use in moderation.

Mustard

Made with ground mustard seeds, mustard has a wonderful color because it is packed with carotenes, lutein, zeaxanthin, and other natural substances that are vital to eye health. Mustard also contains calcium, potassium, phosphorus, magnesium, selenium, B vitamins, and even a little omega-3 fatty acids. Very often, this popular condiment includes turmeric, which has powerful antioxidant, anti-inflammatory, and anti-tumor activity, and has been shown to have eye-protective properties. (See page 79 to learn more about turmeric.)

Although mustard may seem like the perfect condiment, be aware that it is often high in sodium, and in the case of honey mustard, it may include more sugar than you want. So choose your mustard carefully and use reasonable amounts.

Mayonnaise

Mayonnaise is made from oil, eggs or egg yolks, an acidic ingredient such as vinegar or lemon juice, and other flavorings, such as salt and mustard. The oil may be soy, olive, or canola, or the product may use a combination of these ingredients. Whenever possible, opt for olive or canola oil, which are the healthiest choices, and select an organic mayo, which is likely to be made with healthier ingredients. Be aware that mayonnaise has about 100 calories per tablespoon, almost all of them from fat. Even if the fats are healthy, that's a lot of calories for a small amount of food, so use this creamy condiment sparingly.

Salsa

At its best, salsa is the healthiest condiment you can find. Packed with vegetables like tomatoes, bell peppers, and onions; sometimes featuring fruit like pineapple or peaches; and usually flavored with fresh herbs and spices, salsa is high in nutrients and low in calories. (Often, a quarter cup has only about 20 calories, making it a dieter's dream.) Just be sure to read the Nutrition Facts label and avoid products with a lot of sodium. Then, instead of digging into your salsa with greasy chips, scoop it up with fresh vegetables or use it as a sauce with fish or chicken.

HERBS AND SPICES

One of the easiest and best ways to improve the health benefits of your food is to season it with herbs and spices. If you read the inset on page 176, you already know that spices are rich in antioxidants. In fact, both herbs and spices are concentrated sources of all kinds of nutrients that offer amazing benefits. Cinnamon, for example, has been shown to lower blood sugar levels. Black pepper has anti-depressant effects. Cayenne pepper boosts metabolism and has anti-cancer potential. Ginger can treat nausea and has powerful anti-inflammatory properties. Garlic enhances immune function, lowers cholesterol, and reduces blood pressure. Herbs, from basil to parsley, offer essential vitamins A, C, and K, and are packed with polyphenols—antioxidant plant compounds that help combat disorders such as heart disease and diabetes.

An additional benefit of herbs and spices is that they add flavor to food *without salt*. Once you start using these culinary helpers, you'll probably find that you can omit salt or, at the very least, use less. Be aware that many spice companies now offer delicious salt-free blends that you can use in cooking or sprinkle on your foods at the table. These products boost flavor and nutrition while helping you avoid sodium overload. Spices can even be used as a sugar substitute. For instance, cinnamon is a great way to add sweetness to hot cereal or a cup of coffee while boosting your antioxidant intake. You can even add ground cinnamon or cinnamon pieces to ground coffee before brewing for a wonderfully aromatic cup.

BEVERAGES

As you now know, sodas (whether sugar-sweetened or diet), fruit drinks, and sports drinks have no place in your Anti-AMD Diet. Fortunately, you have several healthier choices.

Water is your best option on practically any diet. To put it simply, water is needed for life. When you are dehydrated, your health suffers, as water is essential for proper blood flow, to keep cells plump and healthy, and even for the proper functioning of your eyes. So drink water whenever possible, getting the highest-quality water you can find. If you find a glass of H_2O a little boring, add a squeeze of lemon or lime juice—but no sugar!

Another good beverage choice is tea, especially green tea. Green tea is rich in healthful compounds called catechins, which are disease-fighting antioxidants, and also contains beta-carotene, several B vitamins, vitamin E, several minerals, and a component called theanine, which has been found to lower blood pressure and enhance relaxation. Many of these nutrients are known to protect the delicate tissues of the eye. Moreover, in a study published in the *Journal of Agricultural and Food Chemistry*, catechins were found to penetrate the eye—especially the retina—where they offer protection against cellular damage. The antioxidant activity of the catechins was found to last up to twenty hours. If you're a black tea drinker, rest assured that the theaflavins in black tea are also powerful antioxidants. To keep your tea healthful, use only small amount of the wholesome sweeteners discussed on page 177.

In recent years, studies have shown coffee to offer numerous health benefits, from increased brain activity to the regulation of blood sugar levels. Can coffee also benefit your eyes? More research is needed, but a study performed by Cornell University showed that chlorogenic acid, a strong antioxidant found in coffee, helped protect mice against retina-damaging oxidative stress and free radicals. Just keep your consumption of coffee moderate, and to make your cup of joe as health-promoting as possible, drink it black or use only a tiny bit of the sweeteners discussed on page 177 and a little low-fat milk.

A LAST WORD ABOUT PROCESSED FOODS

Throughout Part Three of this book, we have discussed the problems created by processed foods. Many experts on nutrition believe that processed foods may be the number-one addiction in the United States. The large amounts of sugar, fat, and salt in these foods stimulate the release of the neurotransmitter dopamine, which provides you with a sense of pleasure and reward. Over time, you have to eat more and more of these foods to enjoy the same effects. In the meantime, the foods' unhealthy ingredients—which often include artificial colors and flavors and other additives—are harming your body, including your eyes.

Table 10.3. An Overview of the Anti-AMD Diet

Food Group/ Servings Per Day	Serving Size	Examples	Selected Nutrients Found in Food
Fruits At least 5 servings per day	1 banana, apple, peach, pear, or orange 1 cup grapes or cherries 1 cup cubed melon $1/2$ cup berries	Choose fruits of many different colors—blackberries, blueberries, red apples, red cherries, watermelon, cantaloupe, peaches, citrus fruits, etc.	Vitamins A and C, folate, potassium, fiber, and phytochemicals.
Vegetables At least 5 servings per day	1 cup raw dark green leafy vegetables 1 medium sweet or white potato $1/2$ cup other vegetables 1 cup tomato juice 1 cup vegetable soup 1 cup tomato sauce	Choose vegetables in a wide variety of colors—red and green cabbage, sweet potatoes, squash, dark green leafy vegetables, broccoli, beets, etc.	Vitamins A, C, and K, folate, potassium, fiber, and phytochemicals.
Beans, Peas, and Lentils At least 1 serving per day	$1/2$ cup cooked beans, peas, or lentils 1 cup bean soup	Black beans, black- eyed peas, cannellini beans, chickpeas, (garbanzo beans) edamame, kidney beans, lentils, pinto beans, split peas, etc.	Protein, fiber, B- complex vitamins, calcium, iron, magnesium, potassium, zinc, and phytochemicals.
Nuts No more than 4 servings per week	Small handful of nuts (1.5 ounces) 1 to 2 tablespoons natural peanut or other nut butter	Almonds, Brazil nuts, cashews, hazelnuts, peanuts, pecans, pine nuts, pistachios, etc.	Protein, fiber, essential fatty acids, beta-carotene, B vitamins, vitamin E, calcium, copper, magnesium, phosphorus, selenium, lutein, and zeaxanthin.
Whole Grains 3 servings per day	1 slice bread $1/2$ cup cooked brown rice or other whole grain $1/2$ cup cooked pasta 1 cup ready-to-eat cereal 3 cups popcorn	100% whole grain bread, pasta, or cereal; popcorn; cooked barley, brown rice, quinoa, etc.	Protein, fiber, essential fatty acids, B vitamins, vitamin E, copper, iron, magnesium, phosphorus, selenium, zinc, and phytochemicals.

Poultry, White Meat 2 servings per day *or* 1 serving poultry plus 1 serving fish	3 ounces	Lean skinless white meat chicken or turkey.	Protein, B-complex vitamins, iron, magnesium, phosphorus, selenium, and zinc.
Fish, Preferably Oily 2 to 3 servings per week	3 ounces	Salmon, herring, kippers, mackerel, sardines, trout, and albacore tuna are the best choices.	Protein; vitamins A, B_2, B_6, B_{12}, and D; calcium, iron, magnesium, phosphorus, potassium, sodium, selenium, and omega-3 fatty acids.
Red Meats No more than 1 or 2 servings per week	3 ounces	Lean beef, pork, and lamb.	Protein, vitamins B_6 and B_{12}, iron, niacin, phosphorus, selenium, and zinc.
Eggs 1 serving per day	1 egg	Preferably poached or soft boiled eggs.	Protein; vitamins A, B_5, B_6, B_{12}, and D; choline, lutein, and zeaxanthin.
Dairy Products 2 servings per day	1 cup milk 1 cup yogurt 1.5 ounces cheese	Low-fat milk, low-fat yogurt, low-fat Cheddar cheese, etc.	Protein; vitamins A, D, and B_{12}; calcium, niacin, phosphorus, potassium, riboflavin, selenium, and zinc.
Vegetable oils No more than 2 servings per day	1 tablespoon	Canola, walnut, and olive oil.	Canola oil: Monounsaturated oils, polyunsaturated oils, and omega-3 fatty acids. Walnut oil: Monounsaturated oils, polyunsaturated oils, and omega-3 fatty acids. Olive oil: Monounsaturated oils and vitamins E and K.

Clearly, if the goal of the Anti-AMD Diet is to provide your body with the nutrients it needs to maintain good health and protect your vision, you need to focus on eating whole foods—fresh fruits and vegetables, whole grains, legumes, nuts, lean chicken, and fish. When whole fresh foods take center stage, there's little room left for processed foods, especially highly processed products like snack foods and sugary cereals. When choosing foods like breads, pastas, and cereals, you'll want to look for less-refined options that feature whole grains, as described on page 168. Frozen fruits and vegetables are nutritious convenience foods, so as long as they've been frozen without add-ins such as sugar and salt, you should feel free to include them in your Anti-AMD Diet. Some canned foods—such as canned beans—can also be nutritious and can certainly help speed meal preparation, but again, you have to read the labels and make sure that they don't come loaded down with sodium and other unwanted ingredients. Your ability to read Nutrition Facts labels and ingredients lists (see page 134), will enable you to choose only those foods that will enhance your well-being.

CONCLUSION

You have now learned why the different foods that are part of the Anti-AMD Diet deserve to be on your plate. Table 10.3, found on page 184, provides an overview of the diet by listing the different categories of foods and guiding you toward the proper serving size, the number of servings you can have per day or week, and recommended foods in each group. Finally, the table lists some of the most important nutrients offered by each category of foods.

It's exciting to know that simply by changing your diet, you can not only improve your eye health but also help enhance your overall well-being. Still, change is never easy, and the idea of replacing your current way of eating with the Anti-AMD Diet may be a bit intimidating. Fortunately, the next chapter provides sample meal plans that will ease your transition to your healthier lifestyle. We even include ideas for wholesome snacks and guide you in making wise choices when you're away from home so that you can benefit from the Anti-AMD Diet no matter where you are.

11

℘utting Your Anti-AMD Diet Into Action

I n the last two chapters, you learned about the nutritional components that make foods healthy, as well as the foods that are richest in these valuable nutrients. You also discovered how many servings of each category of food should be eaten and how big each serving should be. (For an overview of the Anti-AMD Diet, see Table 10.3, which begins on page 184.) Now it's time to put all of that information into action.

This chapter begins by reviewing the basics of an eye-healthy diet. We then offer a number of sample menus that show you how to create a day's worth of wholesome meals and snacks. A separate section on snacks guides you in satisfying your between-meals hunger with foods that are packed with nutrients but don't contain the *anti*-nutrients that can sabotage your efforts. Finally, you'll find tips on dining out so that you can enjoy nourishing, health-promoting meals even when you're away from home.

Eating well is a big part of preventing and treating age-related macular degeneration. This chapter will guide you in enjoying a healthy Anti-AMD Diet.

REVIEWING THE BASICS

Following the Anti-AMD Diet isn't difficult, but it does mean organizing meals and snacks so that you get all of the fruits, veggies, lean proteins, whole grains, and other foods that your body needs. It also means avoiding processed foods that are high in salt and sugar and are nutritionally empty. While this may at first seem challenging, the results are worth the effort, because eating the right diet can make an important difference to your vision.

Let's start by reviewing your daily dietary goals. Every day, you should enjoy:

- At least 5 servings of fruit

- At least 5 servings of vegetables

- At least 1 serving of legumes (beans, peas, or lentils)

- Up to 1 serving of nuts (no more than 4 servings per week)

- 3 servings of whole grains or whole grain-based foods

- Up to 2 servings a day of lean skinless white meat chicken or turkey

- Up to 1 serving of fish, preferably an oily variety (no more than 2 to 3 servings per week)

- Up to 1 serving of lean beef, pork, or lamb (no more than 1 or 2 servings per week)

- 1 egg

- 2 servings of low-fat dairy products or dairy alternatives

- Up to 2 tablespoons of organic canola, walnut, or olive oil

Of course, everyone's dietary needs are unique, and you may have one or more health conditions that make it necessary to limit your consumption of certain foods. That's why we believe that it is essential to consult with your doctor or dietitian before you begin the Anti-AMD Diet.

USING THE MENUS

The menus that begin on page 190 guide you in following the Anti-AMD Diet for a full week. Each day's plan includes three satisfying meals plus three nutrient-rich snacks. (See page 197 for a list of snack suggestions.) We've included serving sizes to help you choose healthy amounts of grains, proteins, nuts, dairy products, and oils. When it comes to fruits and vegetables, you can eat as much as you like as long as you have at least five servings of each every day (for a total of at least ten servings) and are able to fit other healthful foods into your meal plan. Fruits and vegetables are very important foods, but you don't want to exclude equally nutritious choices such as legumes, protein, grains, and nuts.

Remember that a serving of vegetables doesn't always have to mean a bowl of salad or a cooked veggie side dish. A cup of vegetable soup, a glass of low-sodium tomato juice, or a ladle of tomato sauce on pasta also counts as a serving. Another option is to incorporate several servings of both vegetables and fruits in a creamy breakfast (or lunch) smoothie.

Naturally, as long as you follow the guidelines provided on page 188, you can replace listed foods with any foods you like from the same category (protein, vegetables, dairy, etc.). But to get the most nutrition out of your meals, do choose the most colorful fruits and vegetables you can find, because those are the ones that are packed with eye-healthy nutrients. If you're not sure which foods offer the greatest benefits, turn back to Chapter 10, "Choosing Foods to Put on Your Plate."

Be aware that the Anti-AMD Diet is a relatively low-calorie meal plan, which can be modified as needed to provide extra calories. Preferably, you should add calories in the form of lean protein, like white meat chicken and fish, and foods rich in healthy fats, like nuts and olive oil. As necessary, provide more generous portions of the most wholesome forms of carbohydrates, such as brown rice, pearled barley, quinoa, beans, and whole grain bread. For additional calories, you can replace low-fat yogurt and cheese with their full-fat counterparts. Another good way to add calories to your menu is to supplement your regular meals with smoothies that combine unsweetened Greek yogurt with fruit and veggies. This will also increase your protein intake. We encourage you to discuss your calorie needs—as well as all of your other nutritional requirements—with your healthcare provider.

DAY 1

BREAKFAST

1 poached egg

1 slice whole grain toast (spread with 1 teaspoon whipped butter or margarine, if desired)

1 orange, cut into segments

1 cup low-fat milk

1 cup coffee or tea

MORNING SNACK

1/2 cup strawberries

1 1/2 ounces walnuts

LUNCH

Turkey sandwich (3 ounces roast turkey on 2 slices whole grain bread with lettuce and 2 teaspoons mustard)

1 cup lentil soup

1 cup red grapes

1/2 cup carrot sticks

1/2 cup cherry tomatoes

1 cup coffee or tea

AFTERNOON SNACK

1 cup plain low-fat Greek yogurt

1/2 cup blueberries

DINNER

1 wedge cantaloupe

3 ounces grilled salmon

1 baked sweet potato

1/2 cup steamed broccoli

Salad made with 1 cup dark leafy greens tossed with 1 tablespoon olive oil and vinegar

1 cup coffee or tea

EVENING SNACK

1 cup low-sodium tomato juice

DAY 2

BREAKFAST	Smoothie made with 1 cup plain low-fat Greek yogurt, 1 cup baby kale, 1 peach, $1/2$ banana, $1/2$ cup fresh pineapple, and 2 teaspoons ground flax seeds
	Toasted whole wheat bagel spread with 2 teaspoons peanut butter
	Coffee or tea
MORNING SNACK	$1/2$ cup blueberries
LUNCH	Salad made with 2 cups romaine lettuce, 3 ounces water-packed albacore tuna, 1 sliced tomato, $1/2$ cup chickpeas, and 1 sliced hard-boiled egg, tossed with $1 1/2$ tablespoons balsamic vinegar and oil
	$1/2$ cup strawberries mixed with $1/2$ cup orange sections
AFTERNOON SNACK	1 apple
DINNER	1 cup cooked spaghetti squash topped with 1 cup tomato sauce made with ground turkey
	1 slice whole wheat bread (spread with 1 teaspoon whipped butter or margarine, if desired)
	1 cup melon balls
EVENING SNACK	1 cup plain low-fat Greek yogurt
	$1/2$ cup fresh raspberries

DAY 3

BREAKFAST	1 cup whole grain ready-to-eat cereal with 1 cup low-fat milk
	1 poached egg
	$1/2$ cup blueberries
	$1/2$ cup orange segments
	Coffee or tea
MORNING SNACK	5 whole grain crackers
	1 $1/2$ ounces low-fat cheese
	1 cup low-sodium tomato juice
LUNCH	Turkey wrap (whole wheat tortilla, 3 ounces roasted turkey, sliced apple, shredded carrots, and 1 tablespoon mayonnaise)
	1 cup bean soup
	1 tangerine
	Coffee or tea
AFTERNOON SNACK	$1/2$ cup cherry tomatoes
	$1/2$ cup broccoli florets
	$1/4$ cup salsa for dipping
DINNER	3 ounces stewed, baked, or grilled chicken
	$1/2$ baked acorn squash with 1 teaspoon olive oil and a sprinkling of cinnamon or nutmeg
	1 cup green beans with caramelized onions
EVENING SNACK	1 peach

DAY 4

BREAKFAST	$1/2$ cup oatmeal with cinnamon and a sprinkling of raisins
	1 cup low-fat milk
	1 peach, sliced
	1 cup coffee or tea
MORNING SNACK	5 whole grain crackers
	1 tablespoon peanut or almond butter
	$1/2$ cup cherry tomatoes
LUNCH	1 cup vegetable soup
	3 ounces chopped cooked chicken breast mixed with 2 teaspoons mayonnaise, herbs, and spices
	$1/2$ cup carrot sticks
	1 banana
	Coffee or tea
SNACK	1 hard-boiled egg
	1 cup red grapes
DINNER	3 ounces grilled or baked salmon
	$1/2$ cup green peas
	$1/2$ cup brown rice
	$1/2$ cup cooked carrots
	Salad made with 1 cup raw kale tossed with 1 tablespoon walnut oil and vinegar
	1 cup mixed fresh fruit
EVENING SNACK	1 apple
	1.5 ounces low-fat Cheddar cheese

DAY 5

BREAKFAST

1 cup low-sodium tomato juice

1 egg, scrambled

1 slice whole grain toast (spread with 1 teaspoon whipped butter or margarine, if desired)

1 cup melon balls, orange sections, and blueberries

Coffee or tea

MORNING SNACK

2 stalks celery spread with 2 tablespoons cashew butter

1 apple

LUNCH

1 cup vegetable soup

1 whole grain pita bread filled with 2 tablespoons hummus, sliced tomato, and sliced cucumber

1 cup red grapes

1 cup low-fat milk

AFTERNOON SNACK

5 whole grain crackers

1 stick low-fat string cheese

DINNER

1 cup turkey chili with beans

Salad made with 1 cup spinach plus 1 cup shredded carrots and purple cabbage tossed with 1 tablespoon olive oil and vinegar

1 slice watermelon

EVENING SNACK

1 cup mixed berries

DAY 6

BREAKFAST

Smoothie made with 1 cup plain low-fat Greek yogurt, 1 cup baby kale, $1/2$ banana, $1/2$ cup fresh pineapple, $1/2$ cup sliced strawberries, and 2 teaspoons ground flax seeds

1 tangerine

Coffee or tea

MORNING SNACK

1.5 ounces walnuts

1 cup red grapes

LUNCH

Egg salad sandwich (2 slices whole grain bread spread with 1 chopped egg, 2 teaspoons mayonnaise, and 1 teaspoon mustard, topped with romaine lettuce)

$1/2$ cup bean salad

$1/2$ cup cherries

1 cup low-fat milk

AFTERNOON SNACK

1 cup carrot sticks, celery sticks, and broccoli florets

$1/4$ cup low-fat vegetable dip

DINNER

3 ounces grilled lean beef

$1/2$ cup quinoa

Salad made with 2 cups dark leafy greens tossed with $1 1/2$ tablespoons olive oil and vinegar

1 cup coffee or tea

1 cup mixed berries

EVENING SNACK

1 cup low-sodium tomato juice

DAY 7	
BREAKFAST	$^1/_2$ cup oatmeal with $^1/_2$ cup blueberries
	1 cup low-fat milk
	1 cup cubed mango
	Coffee or tea
MORNING SNACK	1 hard-boiled egg
	5 whole grain crackers
LUNCH	Salad made with 2 cups romaine lettuce, 3 ounces sliced grilled chicken, $^1/_2$ cup chickpeas, $^1/_2$ cup halved cherry tomatoes, $^1/_4$ cup red onion rings, and 1 $^1/_2$ tablespoons balsamic vinegar and olive oil
	1 apple
AFTERNOON SNACK	1 cup cubed pineapple sprinkled with cinnamon
DINNER	Veggie burger on whole wheat bun with salsa or lettuce and sliced tomato
	Corn on the cob
	$^1/_2$ cup Brussels sprouts, roasted with olive oil and garlic
	1 slice watermelon
EVENING SNACK	1 cup sliced strawberries
	1 cup plain low-fat Greek -yogurt

SMART SNACK IDEAS

If you've read the menus that start on page 190, you've seen that we include three snacks in each day's meal plan. You may have been surprised, because snacking is usually not seen as a beneficial habit—especially since much of the snacking in our country involves greasy salted chips, cookies, ice cream, candy, and the like. Most common snacks are not only nutritionally worthless but also provide health-damaging anti-nutrients like saturated fat, refined sugar, and artificial colors and flavors. Often, they contain a whole day's worth of sodium. Even the best diet can be harmed in a matter of minutes by unwise snacking!

The good news is that snacking doesn't have to be unhealthy. Between-meals snacks can actually help you meet your body's need for fruits, vegetables, and other valuable foods while satisfying your hunger. The following list includes snack ideas from the menus presented earlier, as well as some new ideas. While all of these mini-meals are packed with nutrients, when choosing snacks, it's important to keep in mind the guidelines presented on page 188. It's always a good idea to use snacks to provide needed servings of fruits and veggies, but it's not a good idea to overload your diet with nuts, dairy, or other foods that should be eaten in limited amounts only. So if you spread your morning toast with cashew butter, we don't suggest munching on nuts during the day. We wish you happy and healthy snacking!

❑ 1 slice whole grain bread topped with 1 or 2 tablespoons of peanut, almond, or cashew butter.

❑ 1/2 cup fresh strawberries, blueberries, blackberries, or raspberries.

❑ 1 apple plus a handful of walnuts (about 1.5 ounces of nuts).

❑ 1 cup plain low-fat Greek yogurt, sweetened (if desired) with a small amount of honey or some chopped fresh fruit.

❑ Belgian endives and celery sticks served with 1/2 cup salsa.

❑ Cherry tomatoes and broccoli florets served with 1/4 cup low-fat yogurt-based dip.

❑ 5 whole grain crackers topped with 11/2 ounces of low-fat Cheddar cheese.

❑ 5 whole grain crackers spread with 1 or 2 tablespoons of peanut, almond, or cashew butter.

❑ Carrot and celery sticks served with 1/4 cup hummus or guacamole.

❑ 1 hard-boiled egg plus 1 cup of red grapes.

❑ 1 peach, pear, orange, apple, or tangerine.

❑ 1 stick low-fat string cheese.

❑ 1 cup low-sodium tomato juice or vegetable juice cocktail.

❑ 1/2 cup blueberries plus a handful of almonds (about 1.5 ounces of nuts).

❑ 1 cup steamed or boiled edamame (young soybeans), lightly sprinkled with salt.

❑ 1/2 avocado drizzled with fresh lemon juice or hot sauce.

❑ 1 or 2 unsweetened rice cakes spread with 1 or 2 tablespoons of peanut, almond, or cashew butter.

❑ Half a toasted whole grain English muffin spread with 1 tablespoon peanut butter, thin slices of apple, and a sprinkling of cinnamon.

❑ 3 cups popcorn, preferably air-popped, with a very light sprinkling of salt; Parmesan cheese; or (even better) salt-free herbs and spices.

❑ 1 banana rolled in $1^{1}/_{2}$ ounces of chopped nuts.

❑ 1 cup red grapes frozen into "mini popsicles."

DINING OUT

Eating out can be fun, giving you time spent with friends and family as well as delicious food that you don't have to prepare yourself. But dining out can also throw a wrench into your carefully planned diet. Unfortunately, restaurants generally offer large portions of food that's loaded with salt and fat. But this doesn't mean that you must eat at home to protect your eyesight. Many restaurants offer satisfying choices that are nutritious and will fit into your Anti-AMD Diet, and many are willing to modify their offerings so that you can get what you want. The rest of this chapter offers tips to guide you to the best selections when eating out, enabling you to make the most of menu items in a wide variety of settings.

Inspect the Menu Ahead of Time

Many restaurants either post their menus online or offer printed copies that you can keep on file. This will give you a chance to read through the menu ahead of time and determine if there are any good anti-AMD choices, like salmon or skinless chicken. This will also prepare you to ask questions about ingredients and cooking methods. You can even call ahead of time to make sure that the restaurant is willing to be flexible in the way they prepare your food. By choosing the right restaurant, you will greatly improve your chance of getting food that will work well with your diet.

Be Smart About Portion Sizes

You are probably aware that most restaurants offer oversized portions. The result is that many of us overload on fat, salt, and sugar every time we dine out. The following tips will help you deal with restaurant-size servings.

❑ Ask the server if you can order a smaller portion. Some restaurants are willing to serve a half-size or "senior" portion, usually for a reduced price.

❑ Eat out for lunch instead of dinner. Both portions and prices are substantially smaller at lunchtime than they are at dinnertime, so you can cut down on fat, salt, and sugar while saving money in the process.

❑ Split the entrée with someone, or just take half of it home for another meal.

❑ Create a meal out of appetizers and side dishes, such as a cup of vegetable soup, a shrimp cocktail, and a salad.

❑ Request generous portions of vegetables and salads and smaller portions of chicken, fish, or meat.

Choose the Way Your Dish Is Prepared

Unless the restaurant prohibits any substitutions, you will probably be able to get many foods prepared the way you wish. For instance,

Following a Healthy Anti-AMD Lifestyle in an Assisted Living Facility

If you or a loved one lives in a facility where meals are planned and prepared by others, you can still choose wholesome foods and follow other lifestyle habits that support good eye health. Often, menus are brought around for the next day, giving you a chance to check the healthiest items offered. If a dietitian comes around from time to time, discuss the types of foods you'd like to see on the menus and the ways you would like to have your meals prepared. If foods are served buffet-style in a community dining room, choose a couple of servings of fruits and vegetables at every meal, including breakfast. Select fish, poultry, and—less often—lean meats. Go easy on dessert. If fresh fruit, low-fat yogurt, or low-fat frozen yogurt are available, those would be your best choices.

When family and friends visit, they tend to bring unhealthy snacks like cookies, candies, and cake. Request that they bring fresh fruits and unsalted nuts, unsalted popcorn, or whole grain crackers. Also speak to the facility about providing healthy snacks. Some places pop corn for their residents. Ask if they can also provide cut-up fresh veggies with hummus or salsa for dipping.

Hopefully, you take nutritional supplements—such as the AREDS2 formula—that can help protect your vision. Based upon their location

if they offer fish that's breaded and fried, ask them to poach or grill it instead. Request that French fries be replaced with grilled tomatoes, a green salad, or a side of steamed veggies. You can also request that your salad be served with the dressing on the side. If the restaurant has any whole grain bread on hand, choose it instead of the usual white bread. If the food has not been preseasoned, ask that it be prepared with only a small amount of salt or with no salt at all. Always peruse the entire menu before ordering. Perhaps the salad you want is made with iceberg, but you notice that another salad uses darker greens, like kale, spinach, or romaine. The kitchen should be willing to replace the iceberg lettuce with healthier greens.

Naturally, you will be more successful in protecting your eyes if you order fish and poultry instead of meat. If you must have meat, get

and other factors, assisted living facilities have to follow state and federal guidelines when determining if and how their clients take supplements. Ask the facility if your doctor has to prescribe them even if they are over-the-counter products. Remember that the facility is concerned about possible interactions between your supplements and the other drugs that you are taking, so they need your doctor to make the final decision. You will also want to learn whether you can purchase your own supplements or if the facility has to provide them for you. Finally, you will want to ask if you can take the supplements yourself or if the staff will dispense them.

If you have opportunities to exercise, take advantage of them. You are never too old to engage in some form of light exercise. If physical therapy is available, by all means, take advantage of that, too. The more you move, the better you'll feel, and improved general health usually translates into healthier eyes.

Finally, if AMD is compromising your vision, be sure to take advantage of all the tools available for living with macular degeneration. If the lights in your living area aren't bright enough, have them replaced with brighter lights so that you are able to safely move around, read, or sew. Invest in a good reading lamp made for someone with low vision. Make use of tools such as portable lights and magnifiers. Chapter 13, "Tools for Living with AMD," will guide you to other devices that can help you perform daily tasks and enjoy your favorite hobbies.

the smallest, leanest piece available, or split a larger steak with your dining companion. Then ask for sides that will better support your eye health. Cooked carrots, broccoli, string beans, Brussels sprouts, and baked potatoes (served with a minimum of sour cream or butter, if any) are all good choices. So is a large salad made of greens and veggies. Avoid creamy sauces and cheese toppings.

Anyone who is trying to protect or improve their health should stay away from fast-food restaurants, as they are known for their high fat, high-sodium fare. If you do find yourself at a fast food restaurant, though, look at all the options available and, if possible, choose a green salad, grilled chicken, yogurt, or another wholesome choice. If several burgers are on the menu and you are determined to have one, choose the smallest one that's offered.

Ask for Olive Oil Instead of Butter

Ask that your dishes be prepared with olive oil instead of butter or cream sauces. If your bread is served with butter, ask for a dish of olive oil for dipping. And if the restaurant offers commercial bottled dressings, which are usually not olive oil-based, request cruets of olive oil and vinegar, and drizzle these condiments over your salad. If the restaurant actually makes its own olive oil dressing, always ask that it be served on the side so that you can control the amount added.

Skip or Downsize Dessert

Many of us are no longer hungry by the time we reach the dessert portion of a restaurant meal. If that's true of you, skip the dessert and enjoy a cup of tea or coffee instead. If, however, you find yourself craving something sweet, see if the restaurant is able to provide some fruit—either fresh or poached—or a serving of sorbet. When you simply *must* have a piece of cake or pie, share it with others.

CONCLUSION

The Anti-AMD Diet can be followed at home, when dining out, and even when living in an assisted living facility. That's because there's nothing exotic, unusual, or difficult about this meal plan. As long as you include lots of fruits and vegetables; moderate amounts of legumes, whole grains, nuts, low-fat dairy, and eggs; and small portions of poultry and fish—with only occasional servings of red meat—you will be following an eye-healthy diet.

But, as you probably know, there's more to protecting your eyesight than following a sound diet and taking nutritional supplements. Part Four, "Living Successfully with Macular Degeneration," examines several issues that can make a world of difference to both your vision and your general health.

Part Four

Living Successfully with Macular Degeneration

12

Addressing Lifestyle Risk Factors

In Chapter 3, you learned the risk factors for age-related macular degeneration, which include age, coronary heart disease, gender, genetics, hypertension, inactivity, light exposure, obesity and poor diet, diabetes and prediabetes, race, smoking, and metabolic syndrome. Clearly, some of these factors—age, gender, genetics, and race—cannot be changed. However, all of the other factors can be greatly influenced by lifestyle choices. For instance, diet and exercise can prevent or help control coronary heart disease, hypertension, obesity, diabetes, and metabolic syndrome. The cessation of smoking can decrease your risk of developing these conditions, as well. It all comes down to simple changes that you can make in the way you live your life each and every day.

This chapter looks at a handful of lifestyle changes that can help reduce your risk for AMD. These changes may help you avoid macular degeneration if you do not have the condition. If you have already been diagnosed with AMD, they may be able to stabilize, improve, or even reverse your condition. Just as important, several of these modifications might help you avoid or control other serious health problems, such as heart disease and diabetes.

FOLLOW A HEALTHY DIET
AND MAINTAIN A HEALTHY WEIGHT

Part Three of this book is devoted to helping you adopt the eye-friendly Anti-AMD Diet. Based on extensive research on the relationship between diet and AMD, this eating plan emphasizes abundant portions of fruits and vegetables; moderate servings of whole grains, legumes, and nuts; and limited portions of low-fat dairy, poultry, seafood, and meat. As you learned in Chapters 8 through 11, eating the right foods—and avoiding the wrong foods—can provide your eyes with the nutritional support they need to stay healthy.

The Anti-AMD Diet is a relatively low-calorie diet. By limiting sugar and fat, eliminating junk foods, and keeping portion sizes modest, it can help you shed excess pounds. This is important, as obesity is associated with cardiac disease, diabetes, and many other risk factors for AMD. If you have trouble achieving or maintaining a healthy weight, speak to your physician for advice or enlist the help of a dietitian, who can work with you to create a diet that is appropriate for your health needs.

GET MOVING

The human body is designed to move, so exercise is important for everyone. It is especially crucial, though, for people who are at risk for AMD or have already been diagnosed with it. As you know, exercise is key to preventing and treating heart disease, diabetes, obesity, and other conditions associated with macular degeneration. Moreover, studies have shown that physical activity reduces the chance that you will get AMD or that existing AMD will progress.

Between 1988 and 1990, a study called the Beaver Dam Study—conducted in Beaver Dam, Wisconsin—evaluated men and women between the ages of forty-three and eighty-six and found that physical activity helps protect against wet AMD. The study concluded, "Increased walking of more than 12 blocks daily decreased the incidence of exudative AMD by 30% over 15 years."

A 2003 study was designed to determine what proportion of the elderly population had early or intermediate stages of AMD and what could be done to halt the progression to late-stage macular degeneration. To advise high-risk patients regarding preventive measures, researchers evaluated body type, behavior, and medical factors associated with advancement of the disease. It was found that physical activity decreased the risk for progression to late-stage AMD.

A study in 2009 tested whether the risk of AMD decreases with vigorous physical activity. The researchers found that higher doses of vigorous exercise (running, in this case) were associated with a lower incidence of AMD. These findings were independent of weight, cardiorespiratory fitness, and cigarette use.

The research is clear: Exercise helps prevent and slow the progression of age-related macular degeneration. The studies also show that you will receive benefits whether you engage in vigorous exercise such as running or you simply take long walks. But despite these very encouraging findings, many people avoid physical exercise for all kinds of reasons, including fatigue, disinterest, lack of motivation, and lack of time. Because exercise is so important for your eye health, below we offer some ideas for adding physical activity to your life.

❏ If you haven't exercised in a while, begin at a gradual pace. Start with ten- or fifteen-minute exercise periods, and add five minutes a day.

❏ Add exercise to your sedentary time by using a stationary bike or treadmill as you watch TV or read.

❏ Limit the time you spend on sedentary activities like browsing online or watching TV. If you trim fifteen or twenty minutes from the time you spend sitting still each day, you will find it easier to fit in exercise.

❏ Pick an activity that appeals to you. Take a walk along a beach, dance, or swing a golf club at a driving range.

❏ Avoid monotony by alternating your forms of exercise. Bike through the neighborhood one day, and take a walk through a park the next.

❏ Get an exercise partner with whom you can share your walks, runs, or other activities. It will make your exercise session much more interesting.

❏ Listen to music as you exercise. Music—or perhaps a movie, if you're using home gym equipment—can be a pleasant distraction and make the time pass more quickly.

❏ If you can, hire a personal trainer who can help you exercise safely and keep you motivated.

If you have been diagnosed with AMD and have low vision, you'll want to find a form of exercise that is not just appealing but also safe. Here are a few possibilities:

❏ *Swimming.* This low-impact form of exercise builds endurance and strength. Swim on your own or join an aquatic aerobics class and meet other people with whom you can share the experience.

❏ *Recumbent bike.* Great for cardio workouts, this stationary bike is perfect for people with low vision and is also easy on the joints. Different from a regular stationary bike, it has its pedals at seat height so that it goes extra easy on shoulders, back, and hips.

❏ *Yoga.* A great option for people with low vision, yoga builds strength, muscle tone, endurance, and balance through slow movements. You'll even find yoga mats specially designed for those with low vision. Featuring strategically placed raised and low areas, these mats help you position your hands and feet in the right places.

❏ *Tai Chi.* A Chinese martial art, Tai Chi is practiced for both its defense training and its health benefits. The physical techniques of Tai Chi are characterized by the use of leverage through the joints based on coordination and relaxation, rather than muscular strength. Tai Chi's slow, repetitive motions work to gently and measurably increase circulation throughout the body.

While exercise can make an important difference to your health, if you're older than thirty-five and aren't in the habit of exercising, check with your doctor before starting your new program. This is especially important if you have heart disease, asthma or another lung disease, diabetes, kidney disease, or arthritis. Your doctor can advise you on the types of exercise that are most appropriate for you as well as the recommended duration of your exercise sessions.

STOP SMOKING

As you learned in Chapter 3 (see page 36), studies have shown that smokers are from two to five times more likely than nonsmokers to develop age-related macular degeneration. The more people smoke and the longer they smoke, the higher the risk of the disease. And, of course, according to former Surgeon General C. Edward Koop, cigarette smoking is "the chief, single, avoidable cause of death in our society and the most important public health issue of our time." In other words, even if you're not at high risk for AMD, it's important to avoid this habit. If you are at risk for or already have macular degeneration, it is imperative to stop smoking.

The Eye Disease Case-Control Study Group studied five retinal disorders, including neovascular (wet) age-related macular degeneration. The researchers obtained data from 421 patients with neovascular AMD and 615 control subjects on a wide range of possible risk factors. Smoking was found to triple the risk of AMD. In addition, one of the follow-up reports from the AREDS1 study found a significant association between current and former smokers and more severe manifestations of AMD, including the late stage of dry AMD known as geographic atrophy. In all, about twenty-two studies have shown that smoking correlates to AMD in one form or another.

The suspected mechanism of the disease process is oxidative damage, which is caused by active smoking. The retina is especially susceptible to oxidative damage, and although the carotenoids in the macula work to protect the retina, a 1996 study showed that smokers have less than half the macular pigment density of nonsmokers. Some experts have said that the cessation of smoking is the single most important factor in preventing blindness.

We all know that it isn't easy to stop smoking because nicotine, which is found in all tobacco products, is a highly addictive drug. Nevertheless, every year, about 1.3 million smokers do successfully quit. If you want to quit the habit, consider the various ways of stopping, and choose a plan that you think will work for you. Here are some ideas:

❑ *Cold turkey.* Quitting all at once without outside help is a popular way to stop smoking, but it is not the most effective way: Only about 5 percent of people who use it actually succeed in stopping.

❑ *Behavioral therapy.* This method involves working with a counselor to find your triggers—emotions and situations that make you want to smoke—and to learn to cope with your cravings. According to research, your chance of quitting successfully is doubled when you combine counseling with the right medication.

❑ *Nicotine replacement therapy.* This method works by providing you with nicotine through a means other than tobacco. Instead, you use nicotine patches, gums, sprays, inhalers, or lozenges as you allow your body to adapt to progressively lower levels of nicotine. This method works best when combined with support and behavioral therapy. Patches, gum, and lozenges can be purchased without a prescription, but you will need a physician's prescription for inhalers and nasal sprays.

❑ *Medications other than nicotine replacement therapy.* Prescription medications like bupropion (Zyban and Wellbutrin) and varenicline (Chantix) help you deal with cravings and withdrawal symptoms. Bupropion is an antidepressant that decreases the desire to smoke. Varenicline acts at sites in the brain affected by nicotine, lessening symptoms of withdrawal and blocking the pleasurable effects of smoking. Both are prescription medications.

No matter which method you choose, you will need to create a quit plan in order to succeed. Pick a quit date that gives you time to prepare, and tell family, friends, and coworkers that you intend to give up smoking so that they can provide you with the support and encouragement you need. Then, when it's time to quit, eliminate cigarettes and ashtrays from your home, your car, and your workplace. The goal of protecting your vision should provide you with ample motivation to give up this health-destroying habit.

PROTECT YOUR EYES
FROM DAMAGING BLUE LIGHT

In Chapter 3, we briefly discussed exposure to blue light as a risk factor for AMD. Here we will delve into the issue in a little more detail
so that you will better understand what blue light is, where it comes
from, and how you can provide adequate protection for your eyes.

What we see as "visible light" is actually a small part of the *elec-
tromagnetic spectrum* of energy that is all around us. This energy is
in the form of waves (like ripples on a pond) that emanate from a
source. The waves are in varying energy levels, from short wavelength (high energy) to long wavelength (less energy). Here, we
are concerned with the high-energy blue segment of the spectrum,
which is often referred to as *high-energy visible (HEV)* radiation. The
higher energy wavelengths in the ultraviolet range are absorbed by
the cornea and lens of the eye, so they don't reach the retina. Blue
HEV light, however, penetrates deep into the eye, stressing the rods
and cones and causing them to degrade more quickly. According to
a European study published in the October 2008 issue of *Archives of
Ophthalmology*, blue light may increase your long-term risk of macular
degeneration, especially if you have low blood plasma levels of vitamin C and other antioxidants.

Many eye-care experts are concerned about the potential eye-damaging effects of the blue light that emanates from LED lighting; fluorescent lighting; and computer displays, including laptops, tablets,
and smart phones. However, the most prominent source of this damaging light is the sun. Table 12.1 shows how the blue light found
inside the home and office compares with the blue light that reaches
us through sunlight.

Fortunately, you can take steps to protect your eyes from damaging light; and if you've been diagnosed with AMD, it is important
to take all protective measures available to you. As explained in
earlier chapters, it's vital to eat foods and take supplements that
provide your retina with the lutein, zeaxanthin, and other nutrients
that can help filter out HEV rays. Although computer use has not
been proven to cause AMD, it does typically contain blue light that
can be stressful to the retina. That's why many doctors recommend

Table 12.1. Blue Light Output from Different Sources

Light Source	Blue Power Output (µW/cm²)	Exposure Time Required to Equal 15 minutes in Full Sun
Sunlight	1,000–1,500	15 minutes
LED Lighting	270	1 hour
Compact Fluorescent Lights	38	10 hours
Smart Phone (iPhone 6)	36	10 hours
Computer Screen	30	13 hours
Incandescent Lights	10	38 hours

that you wear protective ophthalmic lenses that have a special coating which filters out the harmful portion of blue light while allowing the harmless portion of the light to pass through. You can also purchase software filters that can reduce the amount of blue light emitted by your display screen. Because less blue light enters the eye, you will find that contrast improves on the computer screen, and eye fatigue is reduced. Specially tinted lenses can also help filter out harmful blue and violet light. Lenses that block blue light are usually yellow in color, but lenses using newer technology are not tinted.

When you're outdoors, sunglasses that are specially tinted or polarized to absorb HEV blue rays will also provide protection for your vision. Be aware that you can't find these glasses on a rack in your local drugstore. Instead, ask your eye-care professional for lenses that block 100 percent of the ultraviolet rays and absorb most HEV rays. Choose sunglasses with a wrap-around close-fitting style, as it will limit the amount of stray light that reaches the eyes from above and beyond the sides of the sunglass lenses. As a bonus, this style offers protection for the delicate skin around your eyes. Small lenses, while they are sometimes fashionable, won't adequately safeguard your vision. Your optician can help you choose the best "blue-blocking" lenses. Many professionals have instruments that can measure the amount of visible light and UV radiation that is blocked by your lenses.

Be sure to wear your blue-blocking sunglasses even when you're sitting in the shade. Although shade reduces your exposure to harmful rays, these rays can still be reflected from buildings, roadways, and other surfaces. On sunny days, fortify your blue-ray defenses by also wearing a wide-brimmed hat. This can reduce your eyes' exposure to ultraviolet and HEV rays by up to 50 percent.

CONCLUSION

In this chapter, we have reviewed some lifestyle issues that can influence the degree to which AMD affects your life. Modifying your lifestyle is not always easy—no one finds it a snap to quit smoking, for instance—but studies show that these changes can offer amazing benefits in terms of better health and vision. And some of the steps you can take, like replacing your current eyewear with blue blue-blocking lenses, are as simple as they are effective.

If you have already lost some vision due to AMD, the changes discussed in this chapter may be able to slow or even reverse the progress of AMD. In addition, there is an ever-growing number of "tools"—from motion-sensing lights to electronic reading devices—that can make it easier for you to function in your everyday life. Turn the page to learn about the devices and techniques that can help you live better with age-related macular degeneration.

$\mathcal{T}$ools for Living with AMD

When age-related macular degeneration progresses to an advanced stage, it can result in a condition known as *low vision*, which means that even with eyeglasses, contact lenses, medicine, or surgery, everyday tasks are difficult to perform. Because AMD affects central vision, many people eventually have trouble reading, driving a car, paying bills, and engaging in other important activities. In more advanced cases, it may even become difficult to walk down a flight of stairs or down a hallway, especially when the lighting isn't adequate.

Fortunately, a variety of tools—from simple magnifiers and lights to more technologically advanced aids—can help you make the most of the vision that remains. Armed with the right devices and techniques, you can often participate in those activities that you need to perform as well as those that provide you with enjoyment.

This chapter looks at several useful low-vision tools as well as some proven techniques that can help you better navigate your world. We will start with modifications that will make it easier for you to perform normal daily activities in your home. We will then look at low-vision enhancements that will help you read and better perform other types of close work, including hobbies, and will even discuss an exciting surgical option. Never have there been more ways to improve your daily life despite low vision.

MAKING IT EASIER TO NAVIGATE YOUR HOME

Just by making a few simple adjustments around your home, you can remove obstacles that may be keeping you from safely moving around your house and carrying out simple tasks. Probably the most important step you can take is to provide better lighting so that you can see, distinguish, and use objects more easily. Fortunately, these days, there are many lighting options available, from super-bright overhead LED lights to small motion-sensing lights that can be easily installed anywhere. While lighting is an important tool, it is not the only tool at your disposal. Contrast is also crucial. By increasing the visual contrast between objects around the house, you will make your life much easier. The following discussions will help you make lighting and contrast work for you.

■ CHOOSE BRIGHT OVERHEAD LIGHTING

A good overhead light—especially in rooms like the kitchen, where you need bright lighting for so many tasks—can be extremely helpful. We suggest purchasing an LED fixture, which produces a bright cool light that is very long lasting. No need to change bulbs! Shop around and choose the highest wattage fixture you can find. Inside many LED fixtures are "arrays." Each array looks like a circuit board and holds many small LED lights. These fixtures provide excellent illumination for large spaces.

Some people prefer halogen lights, which also produce a bright white light. Halogen lights have the advantage of producing less glare, which can be an issue for people with AMD. Although when used as a task lamp, these lights can pose a danger because they reach temperatures so high that they cause burns, this is not a problem when they are used in overhead fixtures.

Another useful option for overhead lighting is the track light, which can be adjusted to illuminate specific work areas. If the space you're working in is large, you will need several track lights—one for each area. These lights are usually incandescent or halogen.

Although overhead lighting is helpful, as AMD advances, it is usually necessary to also provide task lamps for near vision work. That subject is discussed on page 222.

Making Your Morning Cup of Joe

For many years, you may have begun each day with the simple activity of preparing a piping hot cup of coffee. Then your vision began to change, and easy jobs like filling the reservoir with water and measuring out ground coffee became challenging. But you can make this everyday task much less frustrating.

If you don't already have one, invest in a single-serve coffee maker that uses premeasured pods. These devices now come in so many sizes and styles that it should be easy to find one that fits your needs. Some can even produce a whole carafe of coffee to serve a group. Select a color that contrasts with your kitchen countertop. For instance, if you have a dark countertop, get a white or brightly colored coffee maker. Before purchasing the device, make sure that you can easily see and use the controls. By switching to this type of pot, you will be able to skip the frustrating task of measuring out grounds. Moreover, the pods will allow you to make not just coffee, but also tea and hot chocolate. Although you will still have to pour water into a reservoir, you won't have to carefully fill it to a certain mark. Fill the reservoir with a few cups of water, and the machine will automatically measure out the amount of water it needs to make each cup.

Although we urge you to avoid sweeteners, you may not find coffee enjoyable without a touch of sweetness. If so, buy premeasured packets of whatever natural substance you use. (See the discussion of sweeteners on page 177.) Even honey is available in individual plastic packets or tubes, although you may need to order them online.

Do your best to store your pods and coffee mugs in a way that makes them easy to find and identify. Just as you want the color of your coffee maker to contrast with the color of your counter, you want to choose a mug that can be easily spotted and used. These simple changes can make your morning cup of joe as easy to make as it is pleasurable to drink.

■ CONSIDER WEARABLE LIGHTING

Some small lights can be positioned on your body so that you can illuminate an area whenever necessary without searching for a light switch or flashlight. One good option is an LED wrist light. Put it on in the morning and wear it all day so that you can easily find an electrical outlet to plug in your lamp or locate items of clothing in your closet. It should come with an elastic removable strap, be easy to charge, and hold the charge for at least a full day.

A headband light also provides hands-free illumination wherever you go. Choose one that is lightweight and comfortable and features bright LED lights and long-lasting rechargeable batteries.

■ USE MOTION-SENSING STICK-ON LIGHTS

Have you ever wished that your cupboards or closets would light up as you opened them, just as your refrigerator does? Battery-powered motion-sensing lights can be placed anywhere there is a need for better lighting. Position these stick-on devices in linen closets, pantries, clothes closets, and other small dark areas. Some lights can be

---

Understanding Different Types of Lighting

Remember when the lighting in your house and office was either incandescent or fluorescent? Now, so many types of light are available that it takes twenty minutes to choose a light bulb at your local store. If you have AMD, though, it pays to know a little about each form of light. While the following information should help you choose the best fixtures and lamps, remember that everybody's vision is different. You may need to try different types of light bulbs and fixtures before you find what works best for you.

Incandescent Light. Considered the safest light source for your eyes, incandescent light is commonly provided in the form of light bulbs and desk lamps. It is not, however, good for color perception or contrast, nor is it the most economical light available because the bulbs must be replaced frequently.

Fluorescent Light. Most often used in offices and public places, fluorescent light is bright and cost efficient. Modern "compact fluorescent" bulbs provide white light that is bright and safe.

---

connected to a pressure-sensitive switch that turns the light on when the cabinet door is opened. Multi-packs are available for twenty to thirty dollars, making this a relatively inexpensive modification that anyone can install in a matter of minutes.

■ DON'T FORGET YOUR SMARTPHONE LIGHT

Most of us already carry around a handy light—the one on our smartphone! Use the light on your cell phone to help read a menu in a dimly lit restaurant, find the right button on the microwave in your kitchen, read a prescription bottle, use the remote control to your television set, or locate an electrical outlet. Because it is a directed light, this is a great option when overhead lighting or table lamps don't provide the illumination you need and you require a little help for only a short period of time.

Halogen Light. Excellent for enhancing contrast, halogen lighting is bright and white. While it provides a lot of illumination and causes less glare than other forms of light, it is best used in overhead lighting rather than lamps. The heat produced by a halogen bulb is intense enough to burn your hand if you come in contact with it.

LED Light (Light Emitting Diodes). Longer lasting and less expensive to run than any other light source, LEDs provide a bright light without the heat of halogen bulbs. LEDs produce a fair amount of blue light, which has been found to damage the retina in laboratory experiments. However, since you do not stare directly into the light—usually, it's reflected off surfaces into the eye—we consider this light both high in quality and safe.

Full-Spectrum Light. Including the entire range of colors, this form of light is closest to sunlight. Full-spectrum lighting can be very high in blue light, which can damage the retina. Blue light is also responsible for glare, which is a problem for many people with AMD. However, a good-quality full-spectrum light mimics the balance of colors in the sun without the intensity of the sun, making this type of lighting a good choice. Just remember to focus the light on your book or task, not in your eyes.

■ NEVER SKIMP ON LIGHT!

The more light you have in your home, the safer you will be. Add new lamps as needed, and use the highest wattage bulb allowed for each lamp. Replace dark lampshades with sheer white shades that allow more light to enter the room. Provide ample illumination near stairs and in hallways. Consider putting some lights on timers so that important areas of the house are automatically lit as darkness falls. Finally, leave small flashlights and penlights near your microwave, thermostat, washing machine, and any other place where extra lighting may be necessary to see and use controls.

■ USE CONTRAST TO IMPROVE VISIBILITY

Contrast can be as important as lighting in making objects easy to see. Think of how difficult it is to see a black pen on a dark desk. Now replace the black pen with a white one, and see it "pop," enabling you to quickly find it.

You can use the concept of high contrast throughout your home—as well as in outdoor areas—to make objects easier to find and render walking less hazardous. Here are just a few ideas:

- Use dark dishes on a light-colored placemat or white dishes on a black placemat. Another option is to use light-colored plates for dark foods and dark plates for pale foods.

- Select bright, varied colored measuring cups and spoons with large measurement markings.

- When chopping foods, use a dark cutting board when cutting up white potatoes, chicken, and other light-colored foods; and a light cutting board when chopping zucchini, dark leafy greens, carrots, and other brightly colored or dark foods.

- To make electrical switches easier to find, install colored face plates that contrast with the walls of the room.

- In the house, use tape of contrasting colors to outline steps and raised door thresholds.

- Outside the house, paint the edges of steps with white paint.

Large-Type Reading Materials and Electronic Readers

Reading is a challenging activity for most people with advanced AMD. While good task lighting and magnifying devices can help, another option is to simply choose type that is larger and therefore easier to read, or to purchase a device that allows you to easily increase the size of the font, customizing it for your needs.

Large-type books feature not only bigger type but also added space between the lines, which is helpful for people with AMD. Most libraries have a large-type collection, although, of course, it is not as extensive as their regular collection. You can also find large-type books for sale online. Look for used books, as large-type editions tend to be pricey. A number of newspapers—*The New York Times,* for instance—also offer large-type editions that feature selected articles.

An electronic reader allows you to magnify the type to suit your needs and may also enable you to adjust the contrast between the words and the background. This is a far less bulky option than large-type books, and also gives you access to many more titles. E-book readers that are especially helpful for people with AMD include Amazon Kindle Paperwhite, Amazon Kindle, Amazon Kindle Oasis, Amazon Kindle Voyage, Barnes & Noble Nook GlowLight Plus, Kobo Aura H2O, and Kobo Aura One. More are being made available all the time. The electronic books themselves can be purchased and downloaded from a number of sources, the best known being Amazon and Barnes & Noble. Don't overlook your library as a source of e-books. Many offer a number of titles free of charge. Just be aware that although your library may have many electronic books, each one is usually suitable for only one type of e-reader. Contact your librarian for more information as well as directions for downloading books to your e-reader.

Finally, for many years, libraries have offered a range of audiobooks. You are likely to find cassettes, CDs, and MP3 discs. If your eyes get tired when you read or you can't see type clearly even when it's large and amply lit, audiobooks may be your best bet.

MAKING IT EASIER TO READ
AND PERFORM OTHER NEAR VISION TASKS

If you enjoy reading and engaging in other activities that require you to clearly see details, it is important to find ways to continue these pastimes. Lighting and magnification are the two most important reading aids for people with AMD. (Large-type books—another option—are discussed in the inset on page 221.) Below, you will learn about several lighting and magnification options as well as devices that combine the two.

■ CHOOSE APPROPRIATE TASK LIGHTING
AND USE IT CORRECTLY

While a bright overhead light is great for providing general illumination in a room, when you want to read a book, use a sewing machine, or build a model ship, a task lamp is necessary.

It's important to be able to focus a light directly on your reading material or other activity. Lamps with adjustable swing arms and gooseneck lamps are best, because they enable you to move the stream of light to where you need it. To avoid accidental burns, choose a lamp in which the bulb is recessed into the shade. This will also reduce glare. Avoid halogen lamps, which can get quite hot and are better used for overhead lighting. If you pair a lamp with a magnifier, place the lamp so that the light shines *below* the magnifying lens. If the light shines directly on the lens, glare may result.

The following tips should help you use your task lamp to greatest effect.

* Position the shade below eye level so that the light is directed on the task, not at your eyes.

* Direct the light on the task at a 45-degree angle. This will make excess light shine away from your eyes. One way to tell if the position is correct is to place a hand mirror directly on the reading material. If you see a reflection of the light bulb, the lamp is in the wrong position.

* If the light is too bright or is creating too much glare, change its

position. It is safe to place the lamp as close as six inches from the book or task.

- For greatest safety, always use task lamps along with general room lighting. You want to be able to see where you are going when you move away from your task.

■ USE READING MAGNIFIERS

Almost as important as appropriate lighting, magnification is a great aid to reading and other near visions tasks. Most people prefer to have a large area of print magnified rather than just a few words or part of a sentence. Unfortunately, full-page magnifiers are not always the best choice because the larger the area being magnified, the weaker the magnification. Most full-page magnifiers—which are usually thin and cover about 12 by 10 inches—offer at most 2X magnification, meaning that they make print appear twice the original size. If magnifier use is accompanied by good lighting or if your AMD isn't too advanced, this relatively small amount of magnification may be sufficient.

Smaller magnifiers, such as a hand-held magnifying glass, can be more powerful. If you need more than 2X magnification, a smaller magnifier is what you should get. Those with higher magnification, such as 5X, may help by making the words appear clearer and crisper, but the trade-off is that less print is visible. It can also be very tedious to hold a magnifier for any length of time.

Dome magnifiers, which can provide 5X or even 6X magnification, are very useful when you are reading at a desk or table. As the name suggests, these are dome-shaped devices that rest on the page and can be easily made to glide across it. Use them for reading books, newspapers, maps, magazines, or mechanical drawings, or for hobbies like stamp and coin collecting. They are also helpful for reading bills and other documents.

Another option is a stand magnifier, which provides hands-free magnification, allowing you to read for an extended period of time or to enjoy hobbies such as knitting. Some are large enough to fit over a small page, but remember that full-page magnifiers tend to be less powerful than smaller devices.

You may also want to consider a magnifying floor lamp, which provides hands-free use as well as bright (usually LED) light. Often, these lamps have adjustable arms so that you can focus the light on the task at hand. Combination magnifiers and lamps are great for reading as well as a range of hobbies and tasks, such as knitting and sewing. Note that almost any type of magnifier may be available with built-in lighting, combining two powerful aids into one device.

Because different magnifiers are better for different jobs, it is a good idea to purchase several types. Just as you will benefit from having several different types of lighting—both overhead lights and task lamps, for instance—you should have a few magnifiers on hand, including small portable ones that you can take with you when you leave your home. If possible, try them out before making a purchase to test their quality and ease of use.

■ CONSIDER HIGH-TECH READING AIDS

Some reading aids combine different technologies to provide a device that can allow almost anyone to read, regardless of their vision problems. For instance, a desktop video magnifier uses a high-definition camera and a video screen to magnify documents, newspapers, photos, and more. Magnification can be more than 60X, and monitors can be upwards of 20 inches in width, permitting a wide field of view.

Some devices combine video magnification with a text-to-speech feature. A device such as this provides you with a clear image of a magnified document and can also read the document aloud to you.

One relatively sophisticated reading aid pairs a small camera that clips onto the wearer's eyeglasses with a portable computer that fits in the wearer's pocket. The system is able to recognize text in newspaper articles, books, restaurant menus, supermarket packages, smartphone screens, and just about any other surface. It converts the text into clear speech, which the wearer hears through a bone-conduction speaker. This is very different from the reading aids described above because it is highly portable.

Some electronic vision solutions are relatively complex to use, while others offer less complexity so that you can begin enjoying your reading aid right out of the box. Check the resources on pages 249 to 250 to find a device that is a good fit for you.

Consider a Medical Alert System

A good part of this chapter has concerned maintaining safety through the use of lighting, contrast, and other techniques and devices that allow you to better navigate your home and outdoor areas. But no matter how safety-focused and careful you are, falls and other medical emergencies can occur. According to the Centers for Disease Control (CDC), more than one in three adults age sixty-five and older fall in a given year. That's why organizations such as the American Association of Retired Persons (AARP) state that medical alerts are a must.

Some people feel that using a medical alert system means that they have lost their independence, but actually, these devices support an independent lifestyle and provide peace of mind. You can be active in the home and even outside, knowing that help will be available if and when it is needed. How do medical alerts work? In most cases, your home is monitored electronically by a button that you wear on your wrist or around your neck. When you press the button, a radio signal is sent to a base unit, which sends an emergency signal through your phone line to the company that is monitoring you. You are then connected with a trained operator, who sends emergency help to you.

There are a number of medical alert companies from which you can choose, including Medical Guardian, LifeStation, MobileHelp, Medical Alert, ADT Health, and HelpButton. When choosing a system, consider the following:

- **What do you need the system to do?** Do you simply want to be able to call for help in the event of an emergency, or do you also want daily check-ins and other services? Different companies offer different programs.

- **What type of equipment would work best for you?** Is the device comfortable to wear and unobtrusive? Is it waterproof and therefore able to be worn in the shower or bath? Also, what is its range, mobility, and connectivity? Does it include a GPS so that it will protect you anywhere you go?

- **How quickly will the company respond, and who will respond?** Ideally, the response time should be seconds, not minutes, and you should be able to talk to a live person who is available 24/7.

- **What does the system cost?** Look for a company with no extra fees for equipment, shipping, installation, activation, and service and repair. You should pay only ongoing monthly fees, which can range from $25 to $45. Avoid entering into a long-term contract.

  Once you choose and set up a system, be sure to assess how it works for you. If it's not a good fit, switch to a company that can provide the practical protection and peace of mind you need.

HOUSEHOLD OBJECTS DESIGNED FOR LOW VISION

Just as large-type books are a boon to people with low vision who like to read, household items that are large in size, marked in large type, or have the capacity to "talk" can help make nearly every aspect of your daily life easier. Fortunately, a number of companies and organizations—some of which are listed starting on page 249 of the Resources—provide innovative products designed for people with low vision.

If you're simply looking for objects with large labels or displays, you're sure to find plenty of them, including extra large big-digit timers, clearly marked bright-handled measuring cups, large-print computer keyboards, large-digit telephones, jumbo playing cards, large-print wall calendars, and more. "Talking" items include indoor-outdoor talking thermometers, atomic talking clocks with large back-lit displays, talking tape measures, talking calculators, and even talking pill containers, which provide audible guidance when taking medication. Other helpful items are easy-thread sewing needles, knife guards, and liquid level indicators. You're sure to find many more great items in websites, stores, and catalogs that address the challenge of living with low vision.

SMART SPEAKERS AND VIRTUAL ASSISTANTS

While at this time, you may not be able to purchase a voice-controlled device that will cook your morning eggs or take out the garbage, there are several easy-to-use gadgets that can help you in many other ways. Devices like the Amazon Echo with Alexa; the Harmon Kardon Invoke with Cortana; Apple's Siri; and Google Home are revolutionizing the way people obtain information, keep track of their chores and appointments, control their home environments, access entertainment, and much more. Referred to as *smart speakers*, they are wireless speakers that respond to spoken commands by means of a virtual personal assistant (Alexa, for instance).

Initially, setting up these smart speakers requires a computer or mobile device of some sort. Once the device has been set up, though, you can use it completely through voice commands and spoken questions such as; "What is the weather today in Eugene, Oregon?," "Who played Peggy in *The Best Years of Our Lives*?" "Spell the word 'lieutenant,'" "Play Gershwin's *Rhapsody in Blue*," or "Read chapter three of *Big Little Lies*." Your digital assistant will help you without the need to use a difficult-to-read remote control, type your question on a computer keyboard, or flip open a dictionary. Many of these services can also be connected to smart home devices such as lights, thermostats, garage doors, sprinklers, and security systems. This will enable you to dim lights, turn up the heat, and perform other tasks without dealing with light switches and hard-to-read digital displays.

How does your smart speaker know that you're speaking to it and not to someone in the room? In most cases, you activate the unit by speaking the initiation word such as "Alexa" or "Siri." It's that simple. You can use these units in many rooms. For instance, in the kitchen, you might ask your assistant to make a shopping list or to set the timer for fifteen minutes. In the bedroom, you might ask it to set a morning alarm or to play soothing music. Each system provides information and services based on the apps with which it works.

Like all software, the software for digital assistants is getting better all the time, with new skills and updates constantly being incorporated into the programs. If you think you could benefit from a virtual assistant, check the Internet for information on what's available, and be sure to read the reviews written by actual users.

IMPLANTABLE MINIATURE TELESCOPES (IMTS)

As you know, there are few medical treatments available for age-related macular degeneration. However, a new type of surgical implant is offering hope to some people who have lost vision because of this condition.

In 2010, the FDA approved the implantation of a tiny device called an *implantable miniature telescope,* or *IMT.* This device, which is about the size of a pea, magnifies images and projects them onto the healthy areas of the retina, reducing the impact of the central "blind spot" caused by AMD. While this by no means provides perfect vision, about 90 percent of patients experience some improvement, and most have improved facial recognition. In 2012, the IMT became available under a CentraSight treatment program for people with late-stage AMD in both eyes. Medicare covers this treatment for some people.

If you are considered a possible candidate for the IMT, you will be evaluated to see if you are likely to benefit from the implant and, if so, which eye is best suited for treatment. To qualify, you must be seventy-five years of age or older, have stable bilateral (two eyes) end-stage AMD, have evidence of a cataract in the eye considered for the IMT, and be willing to undergo extensive preoperative screening and postoperative training with a low-vision specialist and/or an occupational therapist. Preoperative tests can give you a good idea of what your vision will be like after the implantation.

If you are interested in learning more about IMT surgery, contact your eye-care provider or CentraSight. (Contact information is provided on page 249 of the Resources list.)

KEEPING ON TOP OF NEW BREAKTHROUGHS

Researchers are always developing new technology to help people with vision problems caused by age-related macular degeneration and other conditions. For instance, at this time, a "seeing-eye walking stick" called a Co-Robotic Cane; a smart phone crosswalk app that helps you cross busy streets; a wearable video-based low-vision aid called eSight; and other devices are in the works. Any one of them—perhaps all of them—will eventually provide real help for people with impaired eyesight. When you visit your eye specialist for checkups, always ask if anything new has become available to assist people with AMD. Your doctor should be able to guide you to useful technology.

A great way to keep on top of technological breakthroughs is to set up a Google Alert, which is a customized Google search that automatically informs you by email of news stories and other Internet materials that explore your subject of interest. On page 250 of the Resources, you'll find a link to directions for setting up a Google Alert. When choosing search terms, try to be as precise as possible. If your search is too general, you may end up with too many results to manage. Use quotes around a group of words if you are looking for them together. For instance, you might search for "macular degeneration" or "Co-Robotic Cane." If you find that you are receiving too many or too few Google Alerts, you can always modify your search to make it narrower or broader in scope.

SUPPORT GROUPS

A diagnosis of age-related macular degeneration may leave you feeling very alone. However, considering estimates that in the United States alone, well over one million people have AMD, you are anything but alone! Research has shown that people with AMD who participate in support groups or self-help programs handle things better than people who try to handle everything on their own. It is more than simply encouraging and supportive to interact with people who face the challenges that you are facing. It often enables you to gather valuable information. The people you meet may be able to tell you about good local doctors and clinics, helpful low vision aids, and other important matters.

To find a local support group for people with AMD, call local hospitals, eye clinics, and senior centers. Also look under the "Support Groups" heading found on page 249 of the Resources list.

CONCLUSION

This chapter has guided you to numerous low-vision aids and discussed a variety of techniques for dealing with the problems posed by advanced AMD. Hopefully, you have found some ideas that can make your life easier and allow you to function better. When you combine these aids and techniques with the nutrition and lifestyle suggestions offered in earlier chapters, we feel confident that you will be able to overcome the challenges that come your way and enjoy quality time with family and friends.

Conclusion

I t is not easy to hear a doctor say that you or a loved one has age-related macular degeneration. It is worse still when the doctor tells
you that there is little action you can take to prevent the advancement of AMD other than taking a supplement that has been shown
to slow its progress, but not to stop it. Moreover, this supplement
appears to have no effect in the earliest stage of the disease.

Fortunately, scientific studies—as well as our own personal expe-
riences—have shown that there is much you can do to help prevent
the development of AMD, to slow its advancement, and perhaps even
to halt it in its tracks. This book was written to explain all of the simple
steps you can take to control age-related macular degeneration.

Our first goal in this book was to teach you about AMD—what
it is, how it's treated, and what its risk factors are. We believe that
knowledge is power, and the more you know about AMD, the better prepared you will be to make informed decisions. It is especially
important to understand macular degeneration's risk factors, because
while some, such as age, can't be changed, others can. And by modifying those factors that *can* be changed, you can positively affect your
eye health.

Most people who are diagnosed with AMD soon learn about the
AREDS2 supplements, which have been proven to slow the progress of
the disorder. But what most don't know is that studies conducted after
AREDS2 have shown that many more nutrients can benefit the eyes
in ways that combat AMD. In this book, you have learned about the
powerful nutrients that can help you in the fight against this disease.

Diet is another area that you can use to positively affect your eye health. There is no scientific doubt that a poor diet contributes to numerous disorders, including coronary heart disease, high blood pressure, obesity, diabetes, and metabolic syndrome—the very health issues that are risk factors for AMD. If you can prevent or reverse these disorders through diet, consider the impact you can have on the health of your eyes.

Lifestyle changes are yet another way you can combat AMD. By adding exercise to your life, giving up smoking, and protecting your eyes from damaging light, you can do a great deal to safeguard your vision and, just as important, to support your general health.

Finally, if you are already being affected by AMD, there are many tools and techniques you can use to lead a better life. And most of the tools are inexpensive, readily available, and easy to use.

It is important to acknowledge that the supplements, dietary changes, and other modifications we share in this book may not produce the same results for everyone. Just as a given medication may have the desired effect for one person but not for another, a nutrient may make a big difference for one person with AMD but offer little help to someone else. However, scientific studies have shown that for many people, the changes we suggest do work. It may involve some trial and error, and it will certainly involve some effort, but you can improve your condition. Converting what you have learned into action is not always easy, but ignoring your AMD or letting your doctor deal with it is not the answer. We are not saying that you shouldn't work with your healthcare professional; you certainly should, especially if other health issues, like hypertension or diabetes, are involved. But you, and not your doctor, must take on the responsibility of improving your diet and your life.

Perhaps one day, medical researchers will find a medication that prevents AMD or a procedure that stops it from advancing once it begins. Now, however, the choices offered by conventional medicine are somewhat limited. Our hope is that the information in this book provides you with a number of new and effective ways to beat back what Father Time has thrown in your path. We wish you better health on the journey that lies ahead.

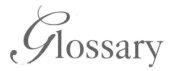

Glossary

This book sometimes uses terms that are common in discussions of eye health and age-related macular degeneration (AMD), but may not be completely familiar to you. You may also hear these terms when working with eye-care specialists. To help you better understand AMD and its treatment, definitions are provided below for words that are often used by those who diagnose and treat AMD, as well as words that are important in this book. All terms that appear in *italic type* are also defined within the glossary.

abdominal obesity. Having a waist circumference that is greater than 40 inches in men and greater than 35 inches in women. This condition is a component of *metabolic syndrome*. See also *obesity*.

acupuncture. An ancient Chinese medical practice that involves the insertion of extremely fine needles to stimulate specific points in the body that assist in healing. Some acupuncturists believe that this practice can improve blood flow to the eye and therefore improve AMD.

advanced glycation end products (AGEs). Compounds formed when sugar molecules in the body latch onto protein or fat molecules, causing a series of transformations. When enough AGEs form, they wreak havoc on the body, resulting in chronic inflammation, hardened blood vessels, and many other health problems.

age-related macular degeneration (AMD). See *macular degeneration*.

alpha-lipoic acid (ALA). A nutrient present in the cells' *mitochondria*, where it is used for energy production. ALA is well known for its *antioxidant* powers and has been shown to protect the mitochondria from *oxidative stress.*

AMD. See *macular degeneration.*

amino acids. The building blocks of *proteins.* There are twenty amino acids. Eleven of them can be made by the body and are considered nonessential because they don't have to be supplied by the diet. The nine amino acids that must be supplied by the diet are considered essential.

Amsler Grid. A grid-pattern chart that is used to determine if images are distorted or if areas of the visual field are missing. This is a standard screening test for AMD and is also used to follow progression of the disease.

anthocyanins. Red, blue, and purple pigments that are found in many fruits and vegetables—including the seeds of red grapes—and provide protection against *oxidative stress* and *inflammation.*

antioxidants. Powerful substances, mostly found in fresh fruits and vegetables, that block oxidation by neutralizing substances called *free radicals,* which otherwise can lead to the dysfunction and destruction of cells. The wide range of antioxidant nutrients includes *beta-carotene,* vitamin C, vitamin E, and selenium.

anti-VEGF drugs. Drugs that inhibit the actions of a protein called *vascular endothelial growth factor* (*VEGF*), which can lead to retinal damage in the wet form of AMD. These drugs include pegaptanib (Macugen), ranibizumab (Lucentis), bevacizumab (Avastin), and aflibercept (Eyelea).

aqueous humor. A clear fluid that fills the small chamber between the *cornea* and the *iris* and provides some nutrition to the adjoining parts of the eye. Also called the aqueous fluid, it flows in and out of the eye on a regular basis.

AREDS. The Age-Related Eye Disease Study, which provided clinical evidence that taking specific supplements reduces the risk of developing advanced age-related *macular degeneration.*

AREDS supplements. Supplements used in the AREDS and AREDS2 studies that have been proven to reduce the risk of developing advanced AMD. These supplements include vitamins C and E, zinc, copper, *lutein*, and *zeaxanthin*.

Best disease. Also known as vitelliform macular dystrophy, a disease that attacks the *macula* and is associated with the buildup of *drusen*. Unlike AMD, Best disease begins to cause changes between the ages of three and fifteen.

beta-carotene. A *carotenoid* that is converted by the body into active vitamin A. Beta-carotene is an excellent *antioxidant* that may help protect the *macula* against *oxidative stress*.

blue light. The high-energy blue segment of the visible light spectrum, sometimes referred to as high-energy visible (HEV) radiation. Instead of being absorbed by the *cornea* and *lens* of the eye, blue light penetrates deep into the eye, stressing the *rods* and *cones* and causing them to degrade more quickly. Some experts believe that blue light increases the long-term risk of *macular degeneration*.

blue-blocking lenses. Eyeglass lenses that filter out damaging *blue light*.

body mass index (BMI). A measure of body fat based on height and weight that applies to adult men and women.

carotenoids. Plant-derived pigments that give plants their bright yellow, orange, and red colors and act as strong *antioxidants* to reduce *oxidative stress*. Carotenoids are important for preventing age-related ailments such as cancer, cataracts, and AMD. There are over sixty carotenoids found in foods, the most famous of which is *beta-carotene*.

central vision. The part of the *visual field* that is directly in front of you and is seen using the *fovea*, which is at the center of the *macula*. In a person with healthy eyes, central vision is the sharpest vision.

choroid. The middle layer of the eye wall sandwiched between the *sclera* and the *retina*. The choroid is filled with blood vessels that deliver oxygen and nutrients to the retina and to other structures found inside the eye.

complete protein. Dietary *protein*, such as chicken and fish, that contains the full complement of *amino acids*, especially the nine amino acids that the body cannot produce on its own and must obtain from foods.

cones. The specialized cone-shaped *photoreceptors* embedded in one layer of the *retina*. Because cones are active in high levels of light and respond to colors, they are essential to daytime vision. Our sharpest vision comes from cones.

conjunctiva. The thin, normally transparent membrane that covers the *sclera* and lines the eyelids.

contrast sensitivity. The ability to distinguish a form from the background or to see subtle changes in the environment. Loss of contrast sensitivity is a sign of AMD.

cornea. The transparent dome-shaped structure that covers the front of the eye. The cornea acts as the eye's outermost lens, functioning as a window that helps focus the entry of light into the eye.

coronary heart disease (CHD). A condition in which a waxy substance called *plaque* builds up inside arteries that deliver oxygen-rich blood to the heart muscle. The buildup of plaque reduces the flow of oxygen to the heart, as well as to the eyes and other organs. That's why there is an association between CHD and AMD.

depth perception. The ability to perceive the relative distance of objects in your *visual field*.

diabetes. A condition characterized by an abnormal metabolism of carbohydrates that leads to elevated blood glucose levels.

diabetic retinopathy. An eye disease caused by *diabetes* in which blood vessel walls are weakened, causing the small blood vessels inside the eye to become more fragile. The blood vessels then leak fluid and blood into the center of the eye, causing loss of vision.

distorted vision. A symptom of AMD in which the damage to the *macula* makes straight lines appear wavy or causes the individual to see shadows or have missing areas of vision. AMD can also cause *impaired color perception* and *impaired depth perception*.

drusen. Yellow deposits of lipids (fats) that accumulate under the *retina*. Although drusen probably do not cause AMD, they indicate an increased risk of developing AMD.

dry macular degeneration. The more common form of *macular degeneration* affecting about 90 percent of AMD patients. It is characterized by the accumulation of *drusen* under the *retina* and blurred or reduced *central vision*.

early AMD. The first stage of AMD, in which it is possible to see small or medium-sized *drusen* scattered throughout the *retina*. Most people do not experience vision loss at this stage.

enzyme. A type of *protein* that is capable of inducing chemical changes in other substances without being changed itself.

epigenetics. The study of mechanisms that switch genes on and off, determining whether or not they get expressed.

essential fatty acids (EFAs). Special dietary fats that are termed "essential" because they are required for good health but cannot be made by the body, and therefore must be consumed in food or supplements. There are two EFA families: *omega-3 fatty acids* and *omega-6 fatty acids*.

fiber. A type of carbohydrate, also referred to as roughage, that is found only in plants and cannot be broken down by digestion and absorbed by the body. There are two types of fiber: soluble and insoluble. Soluble fiber dissolves in water, while insoluble fiber does not.

flavonoids. A large group of *phytochemicals*—with over 6,000 members—that add flavor and color to fruits and vegetables. These nutrients are important in preventing and treating eye disease because of their strong *antioxidant* activity. They convert highly reactive *free radicals* to less reactive free radicals, improve blood flow to the eye, and are anti-inflammatory.

fluorescein angiography. A medical procedure in which fluorescent dye is injected into the bloodstream. The dye highlights the blood vessels in the back of the eye so that it can be determined if the blood vessels are leaking.

fovea. A small dimple found in the middle of the *macula*, where *visual acuity* is the highest.

free radicals. Atoms or groups of atoms with an odd (unpaired) number of electrons. Once formed, free radicals scavenge the body to seek out other electrons to complete the pair. This process causes injury to cells, proteins, and DNA.

full-spectrum light. Light that includes the entire range of colors, making it close to sunlight. Some full-spectrum light is high in *blue light,* which can damage the *retina.*

genetics. The branch of biology that deals with heredity.

geographic atrophy. A late stage of *dry macular degeneration* in which a large portion of the *retina* becomes dysfunctional, causing a loss of vision.

halogen light. A subcategory of incandescent light that produces a bright white light with less glare than many other types of light. The downside is that a light bulb produces a great deal of heat and can burn your hand if touched.

herbalism. The ancient and modern use of leaves, roots, bark, and seeds to prevent and treat various ailments.

high blood pressure (HBP). See *hypertension.*

high-density lipoprotein (HDL) cholesterol. "Good" cholesterol that helps remove "bad" LDL cholesterol from your arteries and recycle it back to the liver.

high-energy visible (HEV) radiation. See *blue light.*

hyperbaric oxygen therapy (HBOT). A therapy in which the patient inhales pure oxygen in a pressurized room or tube. Some practitioners use this as an alternative therapy for AMD.

hyperopia. Far-sightedness.

hypertension. Also called high blood pressure, the flow of blood through blood vessels with higher than normal force. Hypertension is a risk factor for AMD.

impaired color perception. A symptom of AMD in which you have trouble discerning colors, especially in dim lighting conditions.

impaired depth perception. A symptom of AMD that typically occurs when AMD affects one eye more than the other.

implantable miniature telescope (IMT). A tiny device that is implanted in the eye to magnify images and project them onto healthy areas of the *retina.*

inflammation. A reaction of the immune system to harmful stimuli that can include swelling, redness, and pain. Chronic (long-term) inflammation is known to play a key role in age-related disorders such as AMD.

intermediate AMD. The second stage of AMD, in which the *drusen* are typically located in the macular area, and a comprehensive eye exam may detect larger drusen and/or pigment changes in the *retina*. There may be some vision loss at this stage, but there still may not be noticeable symptoms, especially if the changes have occurred in only one eye.

iris. The ring-shaped colored portion of the eye that surrounds the *pupil* and regulates the amount of light that enters the eye. The iris contains muscles that allow the pupil to dilate (open) when there is relatively little light, and constrict (get smaller) when the light is bright.

late AMD. The third stage of AMD, characterized by multiple *drusen* and vision loss from macular damage. Late AMD can be either dry (*geographic atrophy*) or wet (*neovascular AMD*).

LED light (light emitting diodes). A long-lasting energy efficient form of light that produces bright light without the heat of *halogen* bulbs.

lens. Sometimes called the crystalline lens, the resilient, transparent structure behind the *iris* that focuses light on the *retina* by changing the curvature of its front surface.

low vision. A condition in which even with eyeglasses, contact lenses, medicine, or surgery, the degree of vision loss makes everyday tasks difficult to perform.

low-density lipoprotein (LDL) cholesterol. "Bad" cholesterol that contributes to fatty buildup in the blood vessels.

lutein. A *carotenoid* present in certain foods, especially dark leafy greens like kale and spinach. Lutein is one of the three major carotenoids—the others being *zeaxanthin* and *meso zeaxanthin*—that are present in high concentrations in the *macula*. A pigment, lutein helps give the macula its yellowish color and guards the eye from the damaging effects of light, including high-energy *blue light*. Lutein is one of the nutrients included in the *AREDS supplements*.

macula. The central area of the *retina* that is used for sharp, detailed vision, such as that needed for reading and sewing. Together with the *fovea*, it forms the macular region, which is the region that is affected by *macular degeneration.*

macular degeneration. An eye disorder that progressively destroys the *macula*, the central portion of the *retina* that is needed for *central vision*. Macular degeneration is the leading cause of vision loss in adults age fifty and over.

meso-zeaxanthin. One of the three major *carotenoids*—the others being *lutein* and *zeaxanthin*—that are present in high concentrations in the *macula*. Formed by a conversion of lutein in the body, meso-zeaxanthin is not routinely found in the American diet. This pigment guards the eye from the damaging effects of light, including high-energy *blue light*. Meso-zeaxanthin is not included in *AREDS supplements*.

metabolic syndrome (MetS). A cluster of disorders that include *abdominal obesity*, high *triglycerides*, low levels of *high-density lipoprotein ("good") cholesterol, hypertension*, and high blood sugar levels. Sometimes called MetS or Syndrome X, metabolic syndrome is a risk factor for AMD.

microcurrent stimulation. An alternative treatment for AMD in which low levels of electrical current are used to enhance circulation and cellular healing in the *retina* through the use of small probes that are attached to the skin around the eye.

minerals. Naturally occurring substances that are solid and inorganic, meaning that they don't contain carbon. Minerals must be consumed in the diet because the body needs them for important functions but cannot produce them.

mitochondria. Small rod-shaped organs in cells that convert oxygen and nutrients into adenosine triphosphate (ATP), which powers the cells' metabolic activities. For this reason, mitochondria are known as the powerhouses of the cells.

near vision. The eyesight used to see objects that are sixteen inches away or closer. Near vision is needed for reading and other close-up tasks.

neovascular AMD. Also called wet AMD, a type of AMD where weak blood vessels grow below the *macula*, where they leak fluid and blood. This, in turn, results in swelling, damage, and the loss or distortion of vision. Although neovascular AMD affects only 10 to 15 percent of individuals with AMD, it accounts for about 90 percent of all cases of severe vision loss from the disease.

obesity. A condition in which body fat has accumulated to the point where it poses a danger to the individual's health. It is normally defined as a *body mass index* (BMI) of 30 and above. Obesity is a risk factor for AMD. See also *abdominal obesity*.

omega-3 fatty acids. A special class of *essential fatty acids* that includes alpha-linolenic acid, EPA, and DHA. Omega-3 fatty acids play a role in maintaining healthy cell membranes and are anti-inflammatory and antioxidant in their effects.

omega-6 fatty acids. A special class of *essential fatty acids* that includes linoleic acid. Omega-6 fatty acids have many important functions in the body, but if eaten in excess, can have negative effects such as increased inflammation and higher blood pressure.

optic nerve. A nerve composed of the threadlike axons of the ganglion cells (a type of neuron located near the *retina*) that uses electrical impulses to transfer visual information received by the retina to the vision centers of the brain. The two optic nerves (one for each eye) meet in the brain, where the electrical impulses are converted into images.

optical coherence tomography (OCT). A noninvasive procedure that produces cross-sectional images of the *retina* so that the doctor can measure the thickness of the different layers. This can pinpoint areas of the retina that are thinning due to AMD.

optical coherence tomography angiography (OCTA). A noninvasive procedure that generates an image of blood flow to the *retina*.

ORAC. See *oxygen radical absorbance capacity*.

oxidative stress. An imbalance between the production of *free radicals* and the ability of the body to neutralize the free radicals with *antioxidants*. Oxidative stress is associated with many serious disorders, including heart attack, inflammatory disease, and AMD.

oxygen radical absorbance capacity (ORAC). A measure of the effectiveness of the combination of *antioxidants* in a given food at incapacitating a particular *free radical*. The higher the score, the greater the antioxidant action.

peripheral vision. The part of the *visual field* that is outside the direct line of vision; side vision. Peripheral vision is the work of the *rods*, which are largely located outside the *macula*.

photodynamic therapy (PDT). A treatment that uses verteporfin (Visudyne), a light-sensitive drug, in combination with a laser light to eliminate leaking blood vessels that occur in wet AMD.

photoreceptors. Sensory cells found in the *retina* that are stimulated by light. They include the *cones* and the *rods*.

phytochemicals. Chemical compounds produced by plants and commonly found in fruits, vegetables, nuts, legumes, and grains. Some of the better-known beneficial phytochemicals include the *carotenoids*, the *flavonoids*, and resveratrol.

plaque. Fatty deposits that can build up in the arteries, narrowing the arteries and reducing blood flow.

prediabetes. A condition in which blood glucose levels are higher than normal, but not high enough for a diagnosis of fully developed *diabetes*.

presbyopia. Poor *near vision* caused by age-related loss of elasticity of the *lens*.

protein. A nutrient made from *amino acids* that is needed in all body cells for the structure, function, and regulation of body tissues and organs. See also *complete protein*.

pupil. The opening in the center of the *iris* that allows light to enter the eye so it can be focused on the *retina*. The size of the pupil is controlled by the muscles in the iris. One muscle constricts the pupil opening, making it smaller; and another dilates the pupil, making it larger.

retina. A thin layer of tissue that lines the back of the eye. Its purpose is to receive the light that is focused by the *lens*, convert it to neural signals, and send the signals to the brain, where the signals are transformed into an image. The central part of the retina, the *macula*, is the structure that is damaged by *macular degeneration*.

retinal pigment epithelium (RPE). The pigmented membrane found behind the *retina* that is responsible for getting rid of dead cells and for nourishing the nerve tissue of the *macula* and retina.

rods. The specialized rod-shaped *photoreceptors* embedded in one layer of the *retina*. The rods are responsible for vision in low levels of light, and therefore are essential to night vision.

saturated fats. A type of fat, found primarily in animal products, that can raise levels of *low-density lipoprotein (LDL) cholesterol* and place you at higher risk for heart disease.

sclera. The dense white outer covering of the eye that is sometimes known as the white of the eye. Its main purpose is to provide support and protection for the inner eye structures and to attach the eye to the six muscles that control its movement.

Snellen chart. A chart imprinted with rows of letters of different sizes, used to measure *visual acuity.*

Sorsby's fundus dystrophy. An inherited eye disease that causes progressive degeneration of the *macula,* with swelling, bleeding, and pigment changes.

Stargardt disease (STGD). The most common form of inherited juvenile *macular degeneration.*

stereopsis. The depth perception that results from seeing with two eyes. Because AMD typically occurs in one eye before it occurs in the other one, there is sometimes a loss of some depth perception.

trans fats. A type of unhealthy fat made by adding hydrogen atoms to liquid oils so that they become solid like *saturated fats.* Trans fats are more damaging to the health than saturated fats, because they raise levels of *low-density lipoprotein (LDL) cholesterol* but lower levels of *high-density lipoprotein (HDL) cholesterol.* This increases the risk for coronary heart disease, stroke, and type 2 diabetes.

triglycerides. The major form of fat stored by the body. A high triglyceride level increases the risk of heart disease and stroke.

20/20 vision. The *visual acuity* of the optically normal human eye. The term comes from the ability to read a specific row of letters or other symbols on a chart such as the *Snellen chart* from a distance of twenty feet.

ultraviolet (UV) light. Light with a shorter wavelength than visible light but a longer wavelength than x-rays. UV light cannot be seen, but it can cause damage to the eyes and the skin.

visual acuity. The eye's ability to distinguish details and shapes of objects, usually measured by standard eye tests such as the *Snellen chart*. A designation of 20/20 vision indicates what most people call "perfect vision," i.e., you can see at twenty feet what the optically normal eye can see at twenty feet.

visual field. The entire area that can be seen without shifting the position of the eyes. It includes both *central vision* and *peripheral vision*.

vitamins. Organic molecules (meaning that they contain carbon atoms) that must be consumed as part of the diet because they cannot be made by the body.

vitreous humor. A clear gel-like substance that fills the large central chamber of the eye between the *lens* and the *retina*. Because the gel is firm, it helps maintain the spherical shape of the eye and supports the retina. Because it is clear, light can easily pass through it.

wet macular degeneration. See *neovascular AMD*.

zeaxanthin. A *carotenoid* present in certain foods, such as red peppers and carrots. Zeaxanthin is one of the three major carotenoids—the others being *lutein* and *meso-zeaxanthin*—that are present in high concentrations in the *macula*. A pigment, zeaxanthin guards the eye from the damaging effects of light, including high-energy *blue light*. Zeaxanthin is one of the nutrients included in the *AREDS supplements*.

$\mathscr{R}$esources

A number of organizations and websites provide a wealth of information about age-related macular degeneration, its risk factors, its stages, its management, and other topics of interest to the person who seeks to prevent or slow AMD. Directly below, you will find a list of organizations and sites that focus on macular degeneration, as well as one that can assist you in finding research on this disorder. Following this, we offer resources that will help you meet your nutritional needs through good foods and supplements; locate (or start) a support group; find low-vision tools that can improve your daily life; and even set up a computer alert that will keep you abreast of advancements in macular degeneration and its treatments. While we have organized the resources into handy categories, some of these resources provide multiple services—such as presenting information about AMD *and* offering low-vision aids—so it makes sense to visit the various websites and see what each has to offer.

GENERAL MACULAR DEGENERATION INFORMATION

AllAboutVision.com

www.allaboutvision.com /
    conditions/amd.htm

Designed to provide consumers with unbiased information on eye care and vision correction options, this website provides good basic information on a number of conditions, including age-related macular degeneration. You'll learn about the different types of AMD, symptoms and signs, causes, risk factors, and treatments. Click on the link to the Eye Nutrition News page for the latest developments in nutritional research.

American Macular Degeneration Foundation (AMDF)

PO Box 515
Northampton, MA 01061
Phone: 413-268-7660
888-622-8527
Website: www.macular.org

The AMDF serves people who want to learn about and live better with macular degeneration. Their website provides information about the disorder and its treatment; guides you to AMD specialists in your area; informs you of causes and treatments of AMD; and offers a newsletter that includes research updates, healthy living tips, and more.

Bright Focus Foundation

22512 Gateway Center Drive
Clarksburg, MD 20871
Phone: 800-437-2423
Website: www.brightfocus.org / macular

The Bright Focus website provides a Macular Degeneration Toolkit with information about AMD, its symptoms and risk factors, and treatment options. A special page is provided for those who care for someone with AMD.

International Academy of Low Vision Specialists (IALVS)

Phone: 888-778-2030
Website: http://ialvs.com/
The IALVS is a group of optometrists who are specially trained to help patients with low vision, including those with macular degeneration.

Visit this website if you are having problems seeing and performing tasks, and your regular eye doctor says that a change in prescription would not help. The organization's specialists offer a number of low-vision aids, such as spectacle miniature telescopes and implantable miniature telescopes.

Macular Degeneration Partnership

The Discovery Eye Foundation
6222 Wilshire Boulevard, Suite 260
Los Angeles, CA 90048
Website: http://discoveryeye. org /macular-degeneration-partnership/

The Macular Degeneration Partnership provides information and support for people affected by AMD, as well as their family and caregivers. Information is included on diet, low-vision aids, driving, and more. A monthly e-newsletter, available by subscription, presents the latest information about macular degeneration, treatment, and research.

National Eye Institute (NEI)

Information Office
31 Center Drive MSC 2510
Bethesda, MD 20892-2510
Phone: 301-496-5248
Website: https://nei.nih.gov /health/maculardegen/ armd_facts

As part of the federal government's National Institutes of Health, the National Eye Institute has several functions, including the dissemination of health information.

The Facts About Age-Related Macular Degeneration portion of its website offers information about risk factors and symptoms of AMD, treatment options, low-vision services, and support groups. Separate pages are included on important issues such as finding an eye-care professional.

PubMed

Website: www.ncbi.nlm.nih.gov/ pubmed

This search service from the US National Library of Medicine allows you to locate articles from medical literature. Type in the subject of interest, such as "macular degeneration and nutrition," and the titles and authors of hundreds of articles will appear. Click on the ones that sound interesting, and you'll find short summaries. In some cases, you'll

be able to access the complete article without cost. In other cases, your librarian will be able to obtain the articles for you. Just be aware that these are academic articles—not articles written for the general public—and can be difficult to plow through.

WebRN— MacularDegeneration.com

Website: www.webrn- maculardegeneration.com/

Created by a registered nurse who has a family member with AMD, this website was designed to educate people regarding this disorder, including its causes, prevention, and treatments. Topics covered include nutrition, exercise, cutting-edge treatments, low-vision aids, living with AMD, and more.

NUTRITION, SUPPLEMENTS, AND RECIPES

Centers for Disease Control and Prevention—BMI Calculator

1600 Clifton Road
Atlanta, GA 30329-4027
Phone: 800-232-4636
Website: www.cdc.gov/ healthyweight /assessing/bmi/

The CDC provides information on body mass index (BMI), as well as a BMI calculator and information on interpreting the BMI for both adults and younger people.

ConsumerLab.com

333 Mamaroneck Avenue
White Plains, NY 10605

Phone: 914-772-9149 (ext 2)
Website: www.consumerlab.com/

Compiled by an organization independent from supplement manufacturers, ConsumerLab.com offers up-to-date research reports on various nutrients, including vitamins, minerals, and herbs. The site also compares many products by brand, the customary dosage recommended on the label, whether the product contains what the label claims, whether there are any contaminants, and what the price is per daily serving. To gain full access to the site, you must pay an annual subscription fee.

EatingWell

120 Graham Way, Suite 100
Shelburne, VT 05482
Website: www.EatingWell.com

Through its website, the publisher of EatingWell Magazine offers healthy recipes that can be easily adapted for your Anti-AMD Diet.

National Heart, Lung, and Blood Institute (NHLBI)

PO Box 30105
Bethesda, MD 20824
Phone: 301-592-8573
Website: https://healthyeating
   .nhlbi.nih.gov

The Delicious Heart Healthy Recipes section of this website provides wholesome recipes, including some from different ethnic cuisines. Choose dishes with the Anti-AMD Diet in mind—for instance, select chicken rather than beef as a main ingredient—and adapt the recipes as needed.

The Nutrition Source

Harvard School of Public Health
Website: www.hsph.harvard.edu
   /nutritionsource

A product of the School of Public Health at Harvard University, this website offers breaking nutrition news, articles on issues such as sodium and fiber, tips for maintaining a healthy weight, and recipes that can be adapted for the Anti-AMD Diet.

USDA Calculators and Counters

Website: www.nal.usda.gov/fnic/
   calculators-and-counters

Created by the United States Department of Agriculture, this handy website provides links to different calculators, like a body mass index (BMI) calculator; Food-a-Pedia, which provides nutrition information for over 8,000 foods; a Get Moving Calculator, which tells you how many calories you will burn during different activities and exercises; and a Body Weight Planner, which allows you to make personalized calorie and physical activity plans to reach a goal weight and maintain it.

USDA Database for the Oxygen Radical Absorbance Capacity (ORAC Scores)

Website: www.orac-info-portal.de
   /download/ORAC_R2.pdf

Compiled by the United States Department of Agriculture, this website provides the ORAC scores of a range of foods, indicating their antioxidant activity. The higher the ORAC score, the greater the antioxidant action of the food. Included is an introduction that explains the role of antioxidants in maintaining health and an explanation of the procedure used to generate the database.

WebMD Food Calculator

Website: www.webmd.com/diet
   /healthtool-food-calorie-counter

This calculator quickly tells you the calories, fat, carbohydrates, and protein for over 37,000 foods and beverages. It also lets you calculate Daily Totals so you can see how your calories add up.

WebMD How Sugar Affects Your Body

www.webmd.com/diet/features/
how-sugar-affects-your-body

A creation of WebMD, this website will motivate you to break the sugar habit by explaining how sugar adversely affects your brain, mood, teeth, joints, skin, liver, heart, pancreas, kidneys, body weight, and sexual health.

SUPPORT GROUPS

Macular Degeneration Support

www.3600 Blue Ridge Boulevard
Grandview, MO 64030
Phone: 888-866-6148
Website: www.mdsupport.org/
Website for support group: www.
mdsupport.org/support /
international-low-vision-
support-group

The MD Support website provides free information and personal assistance for people dealing with macular degeneration and other retinal diseases. Its International Low Vision Support Group offers extensive online resources,

monthly webcasts, and a public awareness program to reach individuals who are without Internet access.

VisionAware / Support Groups

Website: www.visionaware.org
/info/emotional-support/
peer-support-groups-and-other-
resources/13

The "Support Groups and Other Resources" section of the Vision Aware website provides a list of support groups around the country and gives tips for finding groups in your area or starting your own.

LOW-VISION AIDS

CentraSight

Phone: 877-997-4448
Website: www.centrasight.com

CentraSight offers a treatment program for end-stage macular degeneration that includes implantable telescope technology—a tiny telescope that is implanted in the eye and projects enlarged images onto the healthy area of the retina. Low-vision specialists help you develop the skills you need to use your new vision.

Enhanced Vision

5882 Machine Drive
Huntington Beach, CA 92649
Phone: 714-374-1829
Website: www.enhancedvision
.com

Enhanced Vision offers an extensive line of low-vision aids and electronic magnifiers. Included are transportable magnification units, desk-top video magnifiers with text-to-speech capabilities, and more.

MaxiAids, Inc.

42 Executive Boulevard
Farmingdale, NY 11735
Phone: 800-522-6294 (to order)
631-752-0521 (for information)

Serving people with special needs, MaxiAids is a leading provider of adaptive products, including products designed to make everyday tasks easier for people with low vision. The devices offered through their online catalogue include low-vision clocks, item-identification tools such as talking label readers, large-print items, magnifiers, lighting products, sewing aids, computer accessories, and much more.

OrCam MyEye

1350 Broadway, Suite 1600
New York, NY 10018
Phone: 800-713-3741
Website: www.orcam.com

The OrCAM MyEye is a tiny wearable device that clips onto your eyeglasses. With a camera, a speaker, and a cable that hooks up to a cell phone-size device, this high-tech aid can read whatever you put in front of it—from a newspaper to a can of soup to a ten-dollar bill—and tell you what it says. It also assists in facial recognition by comparing the face in front of the device to previously recorded faces.

SETTING UP A GOOGLE SEARCH

How to Set Up a Google Alert

Website: www.bloggingbasics101
.com/how-to-set-up-a-google-
alert-and-why-its-a-good-idea/

Visit this website to learn to set up a Google Alert. This is a great way to learn about new low-vision aids, including advanced-technology devices, and to make sure that you get breaking information about the treatment of age-related macular degeneration through diet and medicine.

References

Chapter 2. What Is Age-Related Macular Degeneration?

Chaikin L, Kashiwa K, Bennet M, Papastergiou G, Gregory W. Microcurrent stimulation in the treatment of dry and wet macular degeneration. *Clin Ophthalmol.* 2015;9:2345–2353.

Chakravarthy U, Harding SP, Rogers CA, et al. Alternative treatments to inhibit VEGF in age-related choroidal neovascularisation: 2-year findings of the IVAN randomised controlled trial. *Lancet.* Oct 12 2013;382(9900):1258–1267.

Kurok AM, Kitaoka T, Taniguchi H, Amemiya T. Hyperbaric oxygen therapy reduces visual field defect after macular hole surgery. *Ophthalmic Surg Lasers.* May–Jun 2002;33(3):200–206.

Malerbi FK, Novais EA, Emmerson B, et al. Hyperbaric oxygen therapy for choroidal neovascularization: a pilot study. *Undersea Hyperb Med.* Mar–Apr 2015;42(2):125–131.

Owsley C, McGwin G, Jr., Clark ME, et al. Delayed rod-mediated dark adaptation is a functional biomarker for incident early age-related macular degeneration. *Ophthalmology.* Feb 2015;123(2):344–351.

Rofagha S, Bhisitkul RB, Boyer DS, Sadda SR, Zhang K. Seven-year outcomes in ranibizumab-treated patients in ANCHOR, MARINA, and HORIZON: a multicenter cohort study (SEVEN-UP). *Ophthalmology.* Nov 2013;120(11):2292–2299.

Takayama S, Watanabe M, Kusuyama H, et al. Evaluation of the effects of acupuncture on blood flow in humans with ultrasound color Doppler imaging. *Evid Based Complement Alternat Med.* 2012;2012:513638.

Worth ER, Carver JA. Age-related macular degeneration and hyperbaric oxygen. *Undersea Hyperb Med.* Sep-Oct 2010;37(5):375; author reply 376–378.

251

Chapter 3. What Are the Risk Factors for Macular Degeneration?

Adams MK, Simpson JA, Aung KZ, et al. Abdominal obesity and age-related macular degeneration. *Am J Epidemiol.* Jun 01;173(11):1246–1255.

Bhargava M, Ikram MK, Wong TY. How does hypertension affect your eyes? *J Hum Hypertens.* Feb 2011;26(2):71–83.

Cho E, Hung S, Willett WC, et al. Prospective study of dietary fat and the risk of age-related macular degeneration. *Am J Clin Nutr.* Feb 2001;73(2):209–218.

Christen WG, Glynn RJ, Manson JE, Ajani UA, Buring JE. A prospective study of cigarette smoking and risk of age-related macular degeneration in men. *JAMA.* Oct 09 1996;276(14):1147–1151.

Clemons TE, Milton RC, Klein R, Seddon JM, Ferris FL. Risk factors for the incidence of advanced age-related macular degeneration in the Age-Related Eye Disease Study (AREDS). AREDS report no. 19. *Ophthalmology.* Apr 2005; 112(4): 533–539.

Das UN. Diabetic macular edema, retinopathy and age-related macular degeneration as inflammatory conditions. *Arch Med Sci.* Oct 01 2016;12(5):1142–1157.

Fisher DE, Klein BE, Wong TY, et al. Incidence of age-related macular degeneration in a multi-ethnic United States population: the multi-ethnic study of atherosclerosis. *Ophthalmology.* Jun 2016;123(6):1297–1308.

Fraser-Bell S, Symes R, Vaze A. Hypertensive eye disease: a review. *Clin Exp Ophthalmol.* Jan 2016;45(1):45–53.

Hogg RE, Woodside JV, Gilchrist SE, et al. Cardiovascular disease and hypertension are strong risk factors for choroidal neovascularization. *Ophthalmology.* Jun 2008;115(6):1046–1052 e1042.

Hyman L, Schachat AP, He Q, Leske MC. Hypertension, cardiovascular disease, and age-related macular degeneration. Age-Related Macular Degeneration Risk Factors Study Group. *Arch Ophthalmol.* Mar 2000;118(3):351–358.

Loprinzi PD, Swenor BK, Ramulu PY. Age-related macular degeneration is associated with less physical activity among US adults: Cross-sectional study. *PLoS One.*10(5):e0125394.

Mehta S. Age-related macular degeneration. *Prim Care.* Sep 2015;42(3):377–391.

Munch IC, Linneberg A, Larsen M. Precursors of age-related macular degeneration: associations with physical activity, obesity, and serum lipids in the Inter99 eye study. *Invest Ophthalmol Vis Sci.* Jun 06 2013;54(6):3932–3940.

Rudnicka AR, Jarrar Z, Wormald R, Cook DG, Fletcher A, Owen CG. Age and gender variations in age-related macular degeneration prevalence in populations of European ancestry: a meta-analysis. *Ophthalmology.* Mar 2012;119(3): 571–580.

Seddon JM, Willett WC, Speizer FE, Hankinson SE. A prospective study of cigarette smoking and age-related macular degeneration in women. *JAMA*. Oct 09 1996;276(14):1141–1146.

Srinivasan S, Swaminathan G, Kulothungan V, Sharma T, Raman R. The association of smokeless tobacco use and pack-years of smokeless tobacco with age-related macular degeneration in Indian population. *Cutan Ocul Toxicol*. Sep;36(3):253 258

Sun C, Klein R, Wong TY. Age-related macular degeneration and risk of coronary heart disease and stroke: the Cardiovascular Health Study. *Ophthalmology*. Oct 2009;116(10):1913–1919.

Thornton J, Edwards R, Mitchell P, Harrison RA, Buchan I, Kelly SP. Smoking and age-related macular degeneration: a review of association. *Eye (Lond)*. Sep 2005;19(9):935–944.

Chapter 4. Metabolic Syndrome

Cougnard-Gregoire A, Delyfer MN, Korobelnik JF, et al. Elevated high-density lipoprotein cholesterol and age-related macular degeneration: the Alienor study. *PLoS One*. 2014;9(3):e90973.

Ford ES, Giles WH, Dietz WH. Prevalence of the metabolic syndrome among US adults: findings from the third National Health and Nutrition Examination Survey. *JAMA*. Jan 16 2002;287(3):356–359.

Ghaem Maralani H, Tai BC, Wong TY, et al. Metabolic syndrome and risk of age-related macular degeneration. *Retina*. Mar 2015;35(3):459–466.

Hyman L, Schachat AP, He Q, Leske MC. Hypertension, cardiovascular disease, and age-related macular degeneration. Age-Related Macular Degeneration Risk Factors Study Group. *Arch Ophthalmol*. Mar 2000;118(3):351–358.

Imamura F, O'Connor L, Ye Z, et al. Consumption of sugar sweetened beverages, artificially sweetened beverages, and fruit juice and incidence of type 2 diabetes: systematic review, meta-analysis, and estimation of population attributable fraction. *Br J Sports Med*. Apr 2016;50(8):496–504.

Johnson RJ, Nakagawa T, Sanchez-Lozada LG, et al. Sugar, uric acid, and the etiology of diabetes and obesity. *Diabetes*. Oct 2013;62(10):3307–3315.

Khan A, Safdar M, Ali Khan MM, Khattak KN, Anderson RA. Cinnamon improves glucose and lipids of people with type 2 diabetes. *Diabetes Care*. Dec 2003;26(12):3215–3218.

Suksomboon N, Poolsup N, Yuwanakorn A. Systematic review and meta-analysis of the efficacy and safety of chromium supplementation in diabetes. *J Clin Pharm Ther*. Jun 2014;39(3):292–306.

Wang Y, Wang M, Zhang X, et al. The association between the lipids levels in blood and risk of age-related macular degeneration. *Nutrients.* Oct 22 2016;8(10).

Yang L, Colditz GA. Prevalence of overweight and obesity in the United States, 2007–2012. *JAMA Intern Med.* Aug 2015;175(8):1412–1413.

Zhang QY, Tie LJ, Wu SS, et al. Overweight, obesity, and risk of age-related macular degeneration. *Invest Ophthalmol Vis Sci.* Mar 2016;57(3):1276–1283.

Chapter 5. The AREDS Trials

Awh CC, Lane AM, Hawken S, Zanke B, Kim IK. CFH and ARMS2 genetic polymorphisms predict response to antioxidants and zinc in patients with age-related macular degeneration. *Ophthalmology.* Nov 2013;120(11):2317–2323.

Awh CC, Hawken S, Zanke BW. Treatment response to antioxidants and zinc based on CFH and ARMS2 genetic risk allele number in the Age-Related Eye Disease Study. *Ophthalmology.* Jan 2015;122(1):162–169.

Chew EY, Klein ML, Clemons TE, Agron E, Abecasis GR. Genetic testing in persons with age-related macular degeneration and the use of the AREDS supplements: to test or not to test? *Ophthalmology.* Jan 2015;122(1):212–215.

Gorusupudi A, Nelson K, Bernstein PS. The Age-Related Eye Disease 2 Study: micronutrients in the treatment of macular degeneration. *Adv Nutr.* Jan 2017; 8(1):40–53.

Lutein + zeaxanthin and omega-3 fatty acids for age-related macular degeneration: the Age-Related Eye Disease Study 2 (AREDS2) randomized clinical trial. *JAMA.* May 15 2013;309(19):2005–2015.

Parekh N, Voland RP, Moeller SM, et al. Association between dietary fat intake and age-related macular degeneration in the Carotenoids in Age-Related Eye Disease Study (CAREDS): an ancillary study of the Women's Health Initiative. *Arch Ophthalmol.* Nov 2009;127(11):1483–1493.

The Age-Related Eye Disease Study (AREDS): design implications. AREDS report no. 1. *Control Clin Trials.* Dec 1999;20(6):573–600.

Chapter 6. Plant-Based Supplements

Ancillotti C, Ciofi L, Pucci D, et al. Polyphenolic profiles and antioxidant and antiradical activity of Italian berries from Vaccinium myrtillus L. and Vaccinium uliginosum L. subsp. gaultherioides (Bigelow) S.B. Young. *Food Chem.* Aug 01;204:176–184.

Bornsek SM, Ziberna L, Polak T, et al. Bilberry and blueberry anthocyanins act as powerful intracellular antioxidants in mammalian cells. *Food Chem.* Oct 15;134(4):1878–1884.

Broadhead GK, Chang A, Grigg J, McCluskey P. Efficacy and safety of saffron supplementation: current clinical findings. *Crit Rev Food Sci Nutr.* Dec 09 2016;56(16):2767–2776.

Buijsse B, Feskens EJ, Kok FJ, Kromhout D. Cocoa intake, blood pressure, and cardiovascular mortality: the Zutphen Elderly Study. *Arch Intern Med.* Feb 27 2006;166(4):411–417.

Chang YC, Chang WC, Hung KH, et al. The generation of induced pluripotent stem cells for macular degeneration as a drug screening platform: identification of curcumin as a protective agent for retinal pigment epithelial cells against oxidative stress. *Front Aging Neurosci.* 2014;6:191.

Ding EL, Hutfless SM, Ding X, Girotra S. Chocolate and prevention of cardiovascular disease: a systematic review. *Nutr Metab (Lond).* Jan 03 2006;3:2.

Falsini B, Piccardi M, Minnella A, et al. Influence of saffron supplementation on retinal flicker sensitivity in early age-related macular degeneration. *Invest Ophthalmol Vis Sci.* Dec 2010;51(12):6118–6124.

Huynh TP, Mann SN, Mandal NA. Botanical compounds: effects on major eye diseases. *Evid Based Complement Alternat Med.* 2013;2013:549174.

Lashay A, Sadough G, Ashrafi E, Lashay M, Movassat M, Akhondzadeh S. Short-term outcomes of saffron supplementation in patients with age-related macular degeneration: a double-blind, placebo-controlled, randomized trial. *Med Hypothesis Discov Innov Ophthalmol.* Spring 2016;5(1):32–38

Mandal MN, Patolla JM, Zheng L, et al. Curcumin protects retinal cells from light- and oxidant stress-induced cell death. *Free Radic Biol Med.* Mar 01 2009;46(5):672–679.

Marangoni D, Falsini B, Piccardi M, et al. Functional effect of saffron supplementation and risk genotypes in early age-related macular degeneration: a preliminary report. *J Transl Med.* Sep 25 2013;11:228.

Mikkelsen H, Larsen JC, Tarding F. Hypersensitivity reactions to food colours with special reference to the natural colour annatto extract (butter colour). *Arch Toxicol Suppl.* 1978(1):141–143.

Pescosolido N, Giannotti R, Plateroti AM, Pascarella A, Nebbioso M. Curcumin: therapeutic potential in ophthalmology. *Planta Med.* Mar 2014;80(4):249–254.

Piccardi M, Marangoni D, Minnella AM, et al. A longitudinal follow-up study of saffron supplementation in early age-related macular degeneration: sustained benefits to central retinal function. *Evid Based Complement Alternat Med.* 2012;2012:429124.

Richer S, Patel S, Sockanathan S, Ulanski LJ, 2nd, Miller L, Podella C. Resveratrol based oral nutritional supplement produces long-term beneficial effects on structure and visual function in human patients. *Nutrients*. Oct 17 2014;6(10):4404–4420.

Richer S, Stiles W, Ulanski L, Carroll D, Podella C. Observation of human retinal remodeling in octogenarians with a resveratrol based nutritional supplement. *Nutrients*. Jun 04 2013;5(6):1989–2005.

Richer S, Ulanski L, Bhandari A, Popenko N. Longevinex improves human atrophic age-related macular degeneration (AMD) photoreceptor/retinal pigment epithelium mediated dark adaptation. *British Journal of Medicine & Medical Research*. 2017;21(10):1–19.

Ried K, Sullivan T, Fakler P, Frank OR, Stocks NP. Does chocolate reduce blood pressure? A meta-analysis. *BMC Med*. Jun 28 2010;8:39.

Roehrs M, Figueiredo CG, Zanchi MM, et al. Bixin and norbixin have opposite effects on glycemia, lipidemia, and oxidative stress in streptozotocin-induced diabetic rats. *Int J Endocrinol*.2014:839095.

Taubert D, Roesen R, Lehmann C, Jung N, Schomig E. Effects of low habitual cocoa intake on blood pressure and bioactive nitric oxide: a randomized controlled trial. *JAMA*. Jul 04 2007;298(1):49–60.

Tsuruma K, Shimazaki H, Nakashima K, et al. Annatto prevents retinal degeneration induced by endoplasmic reticulum stress in vitro and in vivo. *Mol Nutr Food Res*. May 2012;56(5):713–724.

Wang LL, Sun Y, Huang K, Zheng L. Curcumin, a potential therapeutic candidate for retinal diseases. *Mol Nutr Food Res*. Sep 2013;57(9):1557–1568.

Woo JM, Shin DY, Lee SJ, et al. Curcumin protects retinal pigment epithelial cells against oxidative stress via induction of heme oxygenase-1 expression and reduction of reactive oxygen. *Mol Vis*. 2012;18:901–908.

Yamauchi M, Tsuruma K, Imai S, et al. Crocetin prevents retinal degeneration induced by oxidative and endoplasmic reticulum stresses via inhibition of caspase activity. *Eur J Pharmacol*. Jan 10 2011;650(1):110–119.

Yoon SM, Lee BL, Guo YR, Choung SY. Preventive effect of Vaccinium uliginosum L. extract and its fractions on age-related macular degeneration and its action mechanisms. *Arch Pharm Res*. Jan 2015;39(1):21–32.

Yu CC, Nandrot EF, Dun Y, Finnemann SC. Dietary antioxidants prevent age-related retinal pigment epithelium actin damage and blindness in mice lacking alphavbeta5 integrin. *Free Radic Biol Med*. Feb 01 2012;52(3):660–670.

Chapter 7. Nutrients for Eye Health

Anderson RA, Cheng N, Bryden NA, Polansky MM, Chi J, Feng J. Elevated intakes of supplemental chromium improve glucose and insulin variables in individuals with type 2 diabetes. *Diabetes.* Nov 1997;46(11):1786–1791.

Antioxidant status and neovascular age-related macular degeneration. Eye Disease Case-Control Study Group. *Arch Ophthalmol.* Jan 1993;111(1):104–109.

Beatty S, Chakravarthy U, Nolan JM, et al. Secondary outcomes in a clinical trial of carotenoids with coantioxidants versus placebo in early age-related macular degeneration. *Ophthalmology.* Mar;120(3):600–606.

Belda JI, Roma J, Vilela C, et al. Serum vitamin E levels negatively correlate with severity of age-related macular degeneration. *Mech Ageing Dev.* Mar 01 1999;107(2):159–164.

Broadhurst CL, Domenico P. Clinical studies on chromium picolinate supplementation in diabetes mellitus—a review. *Diabetes Technol Ther.* Dec 2006;8(6): 677–687.

Christen WG, Glynn RJ, Chew EY, Albert CM, Manson JE. Folic acid, pyridoxine, and cyanocobalamin combination treatment and age related macular degeneration in women: the Women's Antioxidant and Folic Acid Cardiovascular Study. *Arch Intern Med.* Feb 23 2009;169(4):335–341.

Delcourt C, Cristol JP, Tessier F, Leger CL, Descomps B, Papoz L. Age-related macular degeneration and antioxidant status in the POLA study. POLA Study Group. Pathologies Oculaires Liees a l'Age. *Arch Ophthalmol.* Oct 1999;117(10): 1384–1390.

Erie JC, Good JA, Butz JA. Excess lead in the neural retina in age-related macular degeneration. *Am J Ophthalmol.* Dec 2009;148(6):890–894.

Erie JC, Good JA, Butz JA, Pulido JS. Reduced zinc and copper in the retinal pigment epithelium and choroid in age-related macular degeneration. *Am J Ophthalmol.* Feb 2009;147(2):276–282 e271.

Evans JR, Lawrenson JG. Antioxidant vitamin and mineral supplements for slowing the progression of age-related macular degeneration. *Cochrane Database Syst Rev.* Nov 14;11:CD000254.

Evans JR, Lawrenson JG. Antioxidant vitamin and mineral supplements for preventing age-related macular degeneration. *Cochrane Database Syst Rev.* Jun 13 (6):CD000253.

Feher J, Kovacs B, Kovacs I, Schveoller M, Papale A, Balacco Gabrieli C. Improvement of visual functions and fundus alterations in early age-related macular degeneration treated with a combination of acetyl-L-carnitine, n-3 fatty acids, and coenzyme Q10. *Ophthalmologica.* May–Jun 2005;219(3):154–166.

Flink EB. Magnesium deficiency. Etiology and clinical spectrum. *Acta Med Scand Suppl.* 1981;647:125–137.

Georgiou T, Prokopiou E. The new era of omega-3 fatty acids supplementation: therapeutic effects on dry age-related macular degeneration. *J Stem Cells*.10(3): 205–215.

Ishihara N, Yuzawa M, Tamakoshi A. Antioxidants and angiogenetic factor associated with age-related macular degeneration (exudative type). *Nippon Ganka Gakkai Zasshi.* Mar 1997;101(3):248–251.

Junemann AG, Stopa P, Michalke B, et al. Levels of aqueous humor trace elements in patients with non-exudative age-related macular degeneration: a case-control study. *PLoS One*.8(2):e56734.

Kook D, Wolf AH, Yu AL, et al. The protective effect of quercetin against oxidative stress in the human RPE in vitro. *Invest Ophthalmol Vis Sci.* Apr 2008;49(4): 1712–1720.

Liang FQ, Green L, Wang C, Alssadi R, Godley BF. Melatonin protects human retinal pigment epithelial (RPE) cells against oxidative stress. *Exp Eye Res.* Jun 2004;78(6):1069–1075.

Michikawa T, Ishida S, Nishiwaki Y, et al. Serum antioxidants and age-related macular degeneration among older Japanese. *Asia Pac J Clin Nutr.* 2009;18(1):1–7.

Millen AE, Voland R, Sondel SA, et al. Vitamin D status and early age-related macular degeneration in postmenopausal women. *Arch Ophthalmol.* Apr;129(4):481–489.

Newsome DA. A randomized, prospective, placebo-controlled clinical trial of a novel zinc-monocysteine compound in age-related macular degeneration. *Curr Eye Res.* Jul 2008;33(7):591–598.

Parekh N, Chappell RJ, Millen AE, Albert DM, Mares JA. Association between vitamin D and age-related macular degeneration in the Third National Health and Nutrition Examination Survey, 1988 through 1994. *Arch Ophthalmol.* May 2007;125(5):661–669.

Qu J, Kaufman Y, Washington I. Coenzyme Q10 in the human retina. *Invest Ophthalmol Vis Sci.* Apr 2009;50(4):1814–1818.

Rosen R, Hu DN, Perez V, et al. Urinary 6-sulfatoxymelatonin level in age-related macular degeneration patients. *Mol Vis.* Aug 21 2009;15:1673–1679.

Sarezky D, Raquib AR, Dunaief JL, Kim BJ. Tolerability in the elderly population of high-dose alpha lipoic acid: a potential antioxidant therapy for the eye. *Clin Ophthalmol.* 2016;10:1899–1903.

Seddon JM, Ajani UA, Sperduto RD, et al. Dietary carotenoids, vitamins A, C, and E, and advanced age-related macular degeneration. Eye Disease Case-Control Study Group. *JAMA.* Nov 09 1994;272(18):1413–1420.

Seddon JM, Reynolds R, Shah HR, Rosner B. Smoking, dietary betaine, methionine, and vitamin D in monozygotic twins with discordant macular degeneration: epigenetic implications. *Ophthalmology*. Jul;118(7):1386–1394.

Shen XL, Jia JH, Zhao P, et al. Changes in blood oxidative and antioxidant parameters in a group of Chinese patients with age-related macular degeneration. *J Nutr Health Aging*. Mar;16(3):201–204.

Simonelli F, Zarrilli F, Mazzeo S, et al. Serum oxidative and antioxidant parameters in a group of Italian patients with age-related maculopathy. *Clin Chim Acta*. Jun 2002;320(1–2):111–115.

Souied EH, Delcourt C, Querques G, et al. Oral docosahexaenoic acid in the prevention of exudative age-related macular degeneration: the Nutritional AMD Treatment 2 study. *Ophthalmology*. Aug;120(8):1619–1631.

Sun YD, Dong YD, Fan R, Zhai LL, Bai YL, Jia LH. Effect of (R)-alpha-lipoic acid supplementation on serum lipids and antioxidative ability in patients with age-related macular degeneration. *Ann Nutr Metab*. 2012;60(4):293–297.

Tao Y, Jiang P, Wei Y, Wang P, Sun X, Wang H. Alpha-lipoic acid treatment improves vision-related quality of life in patients with dry age-related macular degeneration. *Tohoku J Exp Med*. 2016;240(3):209–214.

van Leeuwen R, Boekhoorn S, Vingerling JR, et al. Dietary intake of antioxidants and risk of age-related macular degeneration. *JAMA*. Dec 28 2005;294(24):3101–3107.

Wills NK, Kalariya N, Sadagopa Ramanujam VM, et al. Human retinal cadmium accumulation as a factor in the etiology of age-related macular degeneration. *Exp Eye Res*. Jun 15 2009;89(1):79–87.

Yi C, Pan X, Yan H, Guo M, Pierpaoli W. Effects of melatonin in age-related macular degeneration. *Ann N Y Acad Sci*. Dec 2005;1057:384–392.

Zhuang P, Shen Y, Lin BQ, Zhang WY, Chiou GC. Effect of quercetin on formation of choroidal neovascularization (CNV) in age-related macular degeneration (AMD). *Eye Sci*. Mar 2011;26(1):23–29.

Chapter 8. What *Not* to Put on Your Plate

Amirul Islam FM, Chong EW, Hodge AM, et al. Dietary patterns and their associations with age-related macular degeneration: the Melbourne collaborative cohort study. *Ophthalmology*. Jul;121(7):1428–1434 e1422.

Avena NM, Rada P, Hoebel BG. Evidence for sugar addiction: behavioral and neurochemical effects of intermittent, excessive sugar intake. *Neurosci Biobehav Rev*. 2008;32(1):20–39.

Bokulich NA, Blaser MJ. A bitter aftertaste: unintended effects of artificial sweeteners on the gut microbiome. *Cell Metab.* Nov 04;20(5):701–703.

Chen L, Caballero B, Mitchell DC, et al. Reducing consumption of sugar-sweetened beverages is associated with reduced blood pressure: a prospective study among United States adults. *Circulation.* Jun 08;121(22):2398–2406.

Chiu CJ, Chang ML, Zhang FF, et al. The relationship of major American dietary patterns to age-related macular degeneration. *Am J Ophthalmol.* Jul 2014;158(1):118–127 e111.

Chong EW, Kreis AJ, Wong TY, Simpson JA, Guymer RH. Alcohol consumption and the risk of age-related macular degeneration: a systematic review and meta-analysis. *Am J Ophthalmol.* Apr 2008;145(4):707–715.

Chong EW, Simpson JA, Robman LD, et al. Red meat and chicken consumption and its association with age-related macular degeneration. *Am J Epidemiol.* Apr 01 2009;169(7):867–876.

Ersoy L, Ristau T, Hahn M, et al. Genetic and environmental risk factors for age-related macular degeneration in persons 90 years and older. *Invest Ophthalmol Vis Sci.* Mar 25;55(3):1842–1847.

Ersoy L, Ristau T, Lechanteur YT, et al. Nutritional risk factors for age-related macular degeneration. *Biomed Res Int.*2014:413150.

Farboud B, Aotaki-Keen A, Miyata T, Hjelmeland LM, Handa JT. Development of a polyclonal antibody with broad epitope specificity for advanced glycation endproducts and localization of these epitopes in Bruch's membrane of the aging eye. *Mol Vis.* Jul 14 1999;5:11.

Gao Y, Li C, Shen J, Yin H, An X, Jin H. Effect of food azo dye tartrazine on learning and memory functions in mice and rats, and the possible mechanisms involved. *J Food Sci.* Aug 2011;76(6):T125–129.

Kearns CE, Schmidt LA, Glantz SA. Sugar industry and coronary heart disease research: a historical analysis of internal industry documents. *JAMA Intern Med.* Nov 01 2016;176(11):1680–1685.

Kim Y, Je Y. Prospective association of sugar-sweetened and artificially sweetened beverage intake with risk of hypertension. *Arch Cardiovasc Dis.* Apr 2016;109(4):242–253.

Mares-Perlman JA, Brady WE, Klein R, VandenLangenberg GM, Klein BE, Palta M. Dietary fat and age-related maculopathy. *Arch Ophthalmol.* Jun 1995;113(6):743–748.

McCann D, Barrett A, Cooper A, et al. Food additives and hyperactive behaviour in 3-year-old and 8/9-year-old children in the community: a randomised, double-blinded, placebo-controlled trial. *Lancet.* Nov 3 2007;370(9598):1560–1567.

Obisesan TO, Hirsch R, Kosoko O, Carlson L, Parrott M. Moderate wine consumption is associated with decreased odds of developing age-related macular degeneration in NHANES-1. *J Am Geriatr Soc.* Jan 1998;46(1):1–7.

Pase MP, Himali JJ, Beiser AS, et al. Sugar- and artificially sweetened beverages and the risks of incident stroke and dementia: a prospective cohort study. *Stroke.* Apr 20 2017.

Suez J, Korem T, Zeevi D, et al. Artificial sweeteners induce glucose intolerance by altering the gut microbiota. *Nature.* Oct 2014;514(7521):181–186.

Swithers SE. Artificial sweeteners produce the counterintuitive effect of inducing metabolic derangements. *Trends Endocrinol Metab.* Sep 2013;24(9):431–441.

Walker RW, Dumke KA, Goran MI. Fructose content in popular beverages made with and without high-fructose corn syrup. *Nutrition.* Jul-Aug 2014;30(7–8):928–935.

Zhang YH, An T, Zhang RC, Zhou Q, Huang Y, Zhang J. Very high fructose intake increases serum LDL-cholesterol and total cholesterol: a meta-analysis of controlled feeding trials. *J Nutr.* Sep 2013;143(9):1391–1398.

Chapter 9. What Makes a Food Healthy?

Al-Waili N, Salom K, Al-Ghamdi A, Ansari MJ, Al-Waili A, Al-Waili T. Honey and cardiovascular risk factors, in normal individuals and in patients with diabetes mellitus or dyslipidemia. *J Med Food.* Dec 2013;16(12):1063–1078.

Arnarsson A, Sverrisson T, Stefansson E, et al. Risk factors for five-year incident age-related macular degeneration: the Reykjavik Eye Study. *Am J Ophthalmol.* Sep 2006;142(3):419–428.

Bilsborough S, Mann N. A review of issues of dietary protein intake in humans. *Int J Sport Nutr Exerc Metab.* Apr 2006;16(2):129–152.

Brunzell JD. Use of fructose, sorbitol, or xylitol as a sweetener in diabetes mellitus. *J Am Diet Assoc.* Nov 1978;73(5):499–506.

Cardinault N, Abalain JH, Sairafi B, et al. Lycopene but not lutein nor zeaxanthin decreases in serum and lipoproteins in age-related macular degeneration patients. *Clin Chim Acta.* Jul 01 2005;357(1):34–42.

Chiu CJ, Chang ML, Zhang FF, et al. The relationship of major American dietary patterns to age-related macular degeneration. *Am J Ophthalmol.* Jul 2014;158(1):118–127 e111.

Cho E, Seddon JM, Rosner B, Willett WC, Hankinson SE. Prospective study of intake of fruits, vegetables, vitamins, and carotenoids and risk of age-related maculopathy. *Arch Ophthalmol.* Jun 2004;122(6):883–892.

Chong EW, Robman LD, Simpson JA, et al. Fat consumption and its association with age-related macular degeneration. *Arch Ophthalmol.* May 2009; 127(5):674–680.

Davis DR, Epp MD, Riordan HD. Changes in USDA food composition data for 43 garden crops, 1950 to 1999. *J Am Coll Nutr.* Dec 2004;23(6):669–682.

Field DT, Williams CM, Butler LT. Consumption of cocoa flavanols results in an acute improvement in visual and cognitive functions. *Physiol Behav.* Jun 01 2011;103(3–4):255–260.

Hassinger W, Sauer G, Cordes U, Krause U, Beyer J, Baessler KH. The effects of equal caloric amounts of xylitol, sucrose and starch on insulin requirements and blood glucose levels in insulin-dependent diabetics. *Diabetologia.* Jul 1981;21(1):37–40.

Ma L, Dou HL, Wu YQ, et al. Lutein and zeaxanthin intake and the risk of age-related macular degeneration: a systematic review and meta-analysis. *Br J Nutr.* Feb 2012;107(3):350–359.

Majumdar S, Srirangam R. Potential of the bioflavonoids in the prevention/ treatment of ocular disorders. *J Pharm Pharmacol.* Aug;62(8):951–965.

Marangoni F, Colombo C, Martiello A, Poli A, Paoletti R, Galli C. Levels of the n-3 fatty acid eicosapentaenoic acid in addition to those of alpha linolenic acid are significantly raised in blood lipids by the intake of four walnuts a day in humans. *Nutr Metab Cardiovasc Dis.* Jul 2007;17(6):457–461.

Mares-Perlman JA, Brady WE, Klein R, et al. Serum antioxidants and age-related macular degeneration in a population-based case-control study. *Arch Ophthalmol* 1995 Dec;113(12):1518–23.

Mijanur Rahman M, Gan SH, Khalil MI. Neurological effects of honey: current and future prospects. *Evid Based Complement Alternat Med.* 2014;2014:958721.

Mink PJ, Scrafford CG, Barraj LM, et al. Flavonoid intake and cardiovascular disease mortality: a prospective study in postmenopausal women. *Am J Clin Nutr.* Mar 2007;85(3):895–909.

Yaghoobi N, Al-Waili N, Ghayour-Mobarhan M, et al. Natural honey and cardiovascular risk factors; effects on blood glucose, cholesterol, triacylglycerole, CRP, and body weight compared with sucrose. *ScientificWorldJournal.* Apr 20 2008;8:463–469.

Chapter 10. Choosing Foods to Put On Your Plate

Al-Waili N, Salom K, Al-Ghamdi A, Ansari MJ, Al-Waili A, Al-Waili T. Honey and cardiovascular risk factors, in normal individuals and in patients with diabetes mellitus or dyslipidemia. *J Med Food.* Dec 2013;16(12):1063–1078.

Aune D, Giovannucci E. Fruit and vegetable intake and the risk of cardiovascular disease, total cancer and all-cause mortality—a systematic review and dose-response meta-analysis of prospective studies. *International Journal of Epidemiology.* June 2017;46(3):1029–1056.

Chang CH, Chiu HF, Han YC, et al. Photoprotective effects of cranberry juice and its various fractions against blue light-induced impairment in human retinal pigment epithelial cells. *Pharm Biol.* Dec 2016;55(1):571–580.

Chiu CJ, Chang ML, Zhang FF, et al. The relationship of major American dietary patterns to age-related macular degeneration. *Am J Ophthalmol.* Jul 2014;158(1): 118–127 e111.

Clifford T, Howatson G, West DJ, Stevenson EJ. The potential benefits of red beetroot supplementation in health and disease. *Nutrients.* Apr 2015;7(4):2801–2822.

Cougnard-Gregoire A, Merle BM, Korobelnik JF, et al. Olive oil consumption and age-related macular degeneration: The Alienor Study. *PLoS One.* Jul 2016;11(7): e0160240.

Ersoy L, Ristau T, Lechanteur YT, et al. Nutritional risk factors for age-related macular degeneration. *Biomed Res Int.* 2014;2014:413150.

Gopinath B, Flood VM, Louie JC, et al. Consumption of dairy products and the 15-year incidence of age-related macular degeneration. *Br J Nutr.* May 2014;111(9):1673–1679.

Gopinath B, Flood VM, Wang JJ, Burlutsky G, Mitchell P. Lower dairy products and calcium intake is associated with adverse retinal vascular changes in older adults. *Nutr Metab Cardiovase Dis.* Feb 2014;24(2):155–61.

Meghwal M, Goswami TK. Piper nigrum and piperine: an update. *Phytother Res.* Aug 2013;27(8):1121–1130.

Merle BM, Silver RE, Rosner B, Seddon JM. Adherence to a Mediterranean diet, genetic susceptibility, and progression to advanced macular degeneration: a prospective cohort study. *Am J Clin Nutr.* Nov 2015;102(5):1196–1206.

Ritu M, Nandini J. Nutritional composition of Stevia rebaudiana, a sweet herb, and its hypoglycaemic and hypolipidaemic effect on patients with non-insulin dependent diabetes mellitus. *J Sci Food Agric.* Sep 2016;96(12):4231–4234.

Totan Y, Cekic O, Borazan M, Uz E, Sogut S, Akyol O. Plasma malondialdehyde and nitric oxide levels in age related macular degeneration. *Br J Ophthalmol.* Dec 2001;85(12):1426–1428.

Walt W, Joseph JA, Shukitt-Hale B. Blueberries and human health: a review of current research. *Journal of the American Pomological Society.* 2007;61(3):151–160.

Wang PY, Fang JC, Gao ZH, Zhang C, Xie SY. Higher intake of fruits, vegetables or their fiber reduces the risk of type 2 diabetes: A meta-analysis. *J Diabetes Investig.* Jan 2016;7(1):56–69.

Yaghoobi N, Al-Waili N, Ghayour-Mobarhan M, et al. Natural honey and cardiovascular risk factors; effects on blood glucose, cholesterol, triacylglycerole, CRP, and body weight compared with sucrose. *ScientificWorldJournal.* Apr 20 2008;8:463–469.

Chapter 12. Addressing Lifestyle Risk Factors

Klein R, Lee KE, Gangnon RE, Klein BE. Relation of smoking, drinking, and physical activity to changes in vision over a 20-year period: the Beaver Dam Eye Study. *Ophthalmology.* Jun 2014;121(6):1220–1228.

McGuinness MB, Le J, Mitchell P, et al. Physical activity and age-related macular degeneration: a systematic literature review and meta-analysis. *Am J Ophthalmol.* Aug 2017;180:29–38.

Velilla S, Garcia-Medina JJ, Garcia-Layana A, et al. Smoking and age-related macular degeneration: review and update. *J Ophthalmol.* 2013;2013:895147.

$\mathcal{I}$ndex